THIRD EDITION

CROHN'S
& COLITIS

THIRD EDITION

CROHN'S & COLITIS

Understanding & Managing IBD

Dr. A. Hillary Steinhart
MD, MSc, FRCP(C)

*Medical Director, Mount Sinai Hospital,
Inflammatory Bowel Disease Centre*

Crohn's & Colitis, Third Edition

The author would like to thank Dr. Anne Griffiths of the Hospital for Sick Children, Toronto, Canada, for sharing her knowledge and expertise during the writing of the first edition of this book.

For complete cataloguing information, see page 254.

Disclaimer

This book is a general guide only and should never be a substitute for the skill, knowledge, and experience of a qualified medical professional dealing with the facts, circumstances, and symptoms of a particular case.

The nutritional, medical, and health information presented in this book is based on the research, training, and professional experience of the author, and is true and complete to the best of his knowledge. However, this book is intended only as an informative guide for those wishing to know more about health, nutrition, and medicine; it is not intended to replace or countermand the advice given by the reader's personal physician. Because each person and situation is unique, the author and the publisher urge the reader to check with a qualified health-care professional before using any procedure where there is a question as to its appropriateness. A physician should be consulted before beginning any exercise program. The author and the publisher are not responsible for any adverse effects or consequences resulting from the use of the information in this book. It is the responsibility of the reader to consult a physician or other qualified health-care professional regarding his or her personal care.

Front Cover & Interior Design: Kevin Cockburn/PageWave Graphics Inc.
Back Cover Design & Production: Daniella Zanchetta/PageWave Graphics Inc.
Proofreader: Kelly Jones
Indexer: Gillian Watts
Illustrations: Kveta/Three in a Box
Cover image: Beige textured background © Bill Noll/iStockphoto.com
Back cover image: Balanced white stones © Daniel Chetroni/iStockphoto.com

The publisher gratefully acknowledges the financial support of our publishing program by the Government of Canada through the Canada Book Fund.

Canada

Published by Robert Rose Inc.
120 Eglinton Avenue East, Suite 800, Toronto, Ontario, Canada M4P 1E2
Tel: (416) 322-6552 Fax: (416) 322-6936
www.robertrose.ca

Printed and bound in Canada

1 2 3 4 5 6 7 8 9 MI 26 25 24 23 22 21 20 19 18

Contents

PART 2 • Managing Inflammatory Bowel Disease

Preface

Living with inflammatory bowel disease (IBD) can be a challenge, not only for those of you who have Crohn's disease or ulcerative colitis, but also for those of you who have a family member or close friend afflicted with one of these disorders. Meeting this challenge requires the help of knowledgeable health-care professionals. Knowing what impact Crohn's disease and ulcerative colitis may have on your life and what management strategies are available is also very important. A well-informed patient will have the best chance for recovery and remaining healthy.

However, the amount of information you can find when trying to learn about inflammatory bowel disease can be overwhelming. There are so many possible sources of information — doctors, nurses, books, pamphlets, websites, patient associations, Internet chat rooms, friends, and relatives. Often this information is confusing and contradictory. The quality of the information varies greatly from source to source. This information overload can leave you confused and frustrated, thus making it even more difficult to deal with these chronic diseases.

We have written this book in order to provide patients, families, friends, and health-care professionals with a clear, current, and concise account of the possible underlying causes, clinical features, and effective treatments of Crohn's disease and ulcerative colitis. Rather than simply presenting a list of facts about the disorders, we have given them an applied clinical context based on our years of experience with many hundreds of patients who have been evaluated, followed, and treated at the Mount Sinai Hospital IBD Centre. We have also tried to make this information directly relevant to IBD sufferers and their families by recounting case histories and answering the questions patients frequently ask. We hope to provide another means for dealing with these diseases, which we are only now really beginning to understand.

> We have written this book in order to provide patients, families, friends, and health-care professionals with a clear, current, and concise account of the possible underlying causes, clinical features, and effective treatments of Crohn's disease and ulcerative colitis.

PART 1

UNDERSTANDING CROHN'S DISEASE
AND
ULCERATIVE COLITIS

CHAPTER 1

What Is This Disease?

CASE STUDY Kelly

Kelly, a 22-year-old university student, developed symptoms of abdominal cramping, urgency to move her bowels, diarrhea, and blood in the stool. The symptoms came on gradually and were at first intermittent. They began during the month before her first-term exams, and, although they seemed to improve after she finished the exams, the symptoms continued into the second term. She went to the university health clinic, where she was examined and referred to a specialist. The specialist carried out some tests and told Kelly that she had inflammatory bowel disease, specifically, ulcerative colitis.

Kelly was really upset — ulcerative colitis sounded like a serious disease. Besides, the doctor told her there is no cure, other than surgery. It wasn't fair. "I'm young," she protested, "and no one in my family has had this disease. I've always been very health conscious… I eat a healthy diet, including milk and dairy products. I'm physically active and I don't smoke." She couldn't stop asking questions in her effort to understand why. "What is inflammatory bowel disease? Is colitis an infection? Can I take antibiotics to cure it? Did the stress of my exams cause it? What if I eat a different diet? Could the ibuprofen I take for headaches have an impact?"

Her doctor calmed her down and began answering Kelly's questions…

(continued on page 56)

Inflammation Location

In Crohn's disease, inflammation occurs most often in the lower part of the small intestine, called the ileum, and the large intestine, also known as the colon. Crohn's disease can also affect the esophagus, stomach, and upper parts of the small intestine (duodenum and jejunum).

What Is Inflammatory Bowel Disease?

Inflammatory bowel disease is not a single disease or medical condition. The term describes, in a general way, any condition or disease that results in inflammation of the gastrointestinal tract. Strictly speaking, this definition would include infections of the intestine — for example, infection caused by salmonella bacteria. However, the term "inflammatory bowel disease" (IBD) is usually reserved for two similar disorders, Crohn's disease and ulcerative colitis. Specific causes for these disorders are not yet entirely known.

Crohn's Disease

Crohn's disease probably dates back to the early 19th century, based on descriptions of cases of similar ailments in the medical literature of that era. In 1932, Drs. Crohn, Ginzburg, and Oppenheimer at the Mount Sinai Hospital in New York first described the condition as a specific disease entity. The form of the disease they originally described focused on inflammation of the ileum, the last part of the small intestine. They called the condition regional ileitis, with "ileitis" indicating inflammation of the ileum. Several years after Dr. Crohn and colleagues described the condition, it was given the name Crohn's disease. In the early 1950s, it was recognized that Crohn's disease did not necessarily affect just the ileum, but that other parts of the gastrointestinal tract, such as the colon or large intestine, could be affected.

Ulcerative Colitis

Like Crohn's disease, ulcerative colitis had probably been with us for some time before it was fully described in the late 19th century. Ulcerative colitis is sometimes referred to as ulcerative proctitis, ulcerative proctosigmoiditis, or ulcerative pancolitis. These names relate primarily to the extent of the inflammation of the colon rather than to any fundamental differences in the presumed causes of ulcerative colitis. In the first half of the 20th century, the treatment of ulcerative colitis was surgical, and many patients ended up dying of complications of the disease or the surgery. Since the 1940s, there has been a consistent improvement in the surgical and medical management of ulcerative colitis, and death due to complications of the disease or its treatment is now exceedingly rare.

> **Limited Inflammation**
>
> In ulcerative colitis, the inflammation is limited to the large intestine, which includes the rectum. The rest of the gastrointestinal tract is not involved.

Irritable Bowel Syndrome

Inflammatory bowel disease (IBD) and irritable bowel syndrome (IBS) are often confused since their names are so alike. IBS is a poorly understood condition of the gastrointestinal tract. Although IBS is characterized by chronic abdominal discomfort or pain and an alteration in the normal bowel habit, it is quite a different condition from Crohn's disease and ulcerative colitis (IBD).

In IBS, it is thought that the problems arise from a change in the way the bowel functions or the way in which the brain senses the bowel functioning. In IBS, there has been no clear or consistent evidence that inflammation plays a role in causing the symptoms in humans. This is different from IBD, where inflammation is the main defining characteristic of the disease, and where treatment against inflammation will help treat the disease and alleviate its symptoms. In IBS, treatment is usually aimed at modifying the motility of the gastrointestinal tract or the transmission of the pain impulses from the intestine to the brain.

Glossary of Inflammatory Bowel Disease

Gastroenterologists use several technical terms to describe IBD. You can start to use the language of this disease in discussions with your health-care providers. These terms are defined more thoroughly in their context later in the book.

Abscess: a localized collection of dead and infected tissue (pus), which typically becomes liquid. The consequences may be serious if it is not quickly and properly managed; management involves draining the infected material and treating with antibiotics.

Absorption: the digestive process of extracting nutrients from food and transferring these nutrients into the circulatory system; for example, the absorption of vitamin B_{12} occurs in the ileum (the last section of the small intestine), which is often problematic in IBD.

Anal sphincter: a muscular valve at the bottom of the rectum, which normally prevents stool from coming out when it is not supposed to. Damage to the sphincter or the nerves supplying the sphincter can lead to fecal incontinence.

Colon (large intestine): the lower part of the gastrointestinal tract, which is primarily responsible for reabsorbing fluid and electrolytes (salts) from the stool.

Colonoscopy: a diagnostic procedure for IBD that involves inserting a scope through the anus and rectum to the colon, where a tissue biopsy may be taken for testing.

Distension: a significant increase in the size of the abdomen that may be due to gas, stool, or fluid.

Duodenum: the first part of the small intestine, which receives ingested food after it has left the stomach. Although the duodenum is relatively short (about 12 inches/30 cm in length), it has an important role in the absorption of some nutrients, particularly iron; it is also the location where digestive enzymes from the pancreas and bile salts from the liver are first mixed together with food in order to help the digestion process.

Enzyme: a protein that helps the rate of a chemical reaction, usually related to an important metabolic function of the body.

Fecal incontinence: loss of the ability to hold stool (fecal waste). This may happen when there is inflammation of the rectum or lower part of the colon, or when there has been damage to the anal sphincter.

Fistula: an abnormal communication or channel from the intestine to other organs or to the abdominal wall or skin.

Gastroenterology: a medical specialty involved in the study of the digestive system, digestive disease, and digestive health.

Gastrointestinal (GI) tract: the tract that extends from the mouth to the anus.

Granuloma: a distinctive collection of inflammatory or immune cells that occurs in tissues affected by certain conditions, including Crohn's disease.

Ileum: the last part of the small intestine; it makes up about one-third of the entire length of the small intestine. Vitamin B_{12} is absorbed here.

Inflammatory bowel disease (IBD): any condition or disease that results in inflammation of the gastrointestinal tract, most commonly in the small and large intestine and the rectum.

Irritable bowel syndrome (IBS): a functional GI syndrome characterized by symptoms of abdominal pain or discomfort, along with a change in the bowel habit. There is no inflammation of the GI tract.

Jejunum: the second part of the small intestine, which makes up about two-thirds of the entire length of the small intestine and is responsible for the absorption of most of the nutrients from food.

Lymphocyte: a type of white blood cell that is important in immune protection against a number of different possible bacteria and viruses that can cause infection.

Motility: the movement of food through the GI tract.

Mucosa: the inner lining of the gastrointestinal tract. The integrity of the mucosa is important for carrying out many of the roles of the gastrointestinal tract, particularly digestion of food and absorption of nutrients.

Pancolitis: inflammation that involves the entire colon.

Perforation: a hole in the wall of the intestine, which allows intestinal contents, often with numerous bacteria, into the abdominal cavity, where serious infection may result.

Peristalsis: the involuntary contractions that move food through the GI tract.

Proctitis: a form of colitis that affects only the rectum.

Proteins: compounds made up of long chains of amino acids. Proteins are responsible for many critical functions, including maintenance of bodily structure and metabolic functions.

Rectum: the very last part of the colon (large intestine), where stool is held before it is expelled. Inflammation of the rectum can result in difficulty holding stool for extended periods of time.

Serosa: the outer lining (membrane) that covers the intestine.

Stricture: a narrowing of the central channel in a segment of the intestine, which can lead to obstruction or blockage.

Ulcer: an area in the gastrointestinal tract where there is a loss of the normal internal lining (mucosa). Ulcers can result in complications, such as bleeding or abscesses.

Villi: fingerlike projections of the inner lining of the small intestine (mucosa), which have the effect of increasing the amount of mucosal surface available for absorption of nutrients.

Smoking Paradox

Smoking increases the risk of developing Crohn's disease, and in those already affected, smoking may make the disease more aggressive or severe. In contrast, smoking seems to protect against ulcerative colitis. Patients with ulcerative colitis are more likely to be nonsmokers or former smokers than a similar group of people selected from the general population. In former smokers, the period soon after smoking cessation seems to be a time of particularly increased risk of developing ulcerative colitis. This observation has led some researchers to use nicotine, in the form of skin patches, as a treatment for ulcerative colitis. Despite the strong association between cigarette smoking and protection against ulcerative colitis, this approach to treatment has not been consistently effective.

Who Gets Inflammatory Bowel Disease?

The onset of inflammatory bowel disease may be influenced by age, gender, and geography.

Age Factors

Crohn's disease and ulcerative colitis most commonly begin in young people. Although it is unusual to see this disorder in children below the age of 5, there is an increase in the occurrence of IBD up until the age of 20, with maximum incidence in the age group between 20 and 40. It is less common, but certainly not unheard of, for older individuals in their 50s and 60s to first experience IBD. The first onset of disease is quite rare in the elderly. When symptoms first occur in someone from that age group, the attending doctor will usually consider other conditions or illnesses as more likely than IBD.

Gender

Inflammatory bowel disease appears to occur in males and females at roughly the same rate, although some studies have suggested that there may be slightly higher incidence in females. These differences may vary depending on the age of the first onset of IBD, but even if such differences exist, they are likely to be minor and of no major significance.

Population Studies

Although they are generally thought to be diseases that are found more frequently in developed countries, Crohn's disease and ulcerative colitis have been observed in every race and in every country that has been specifically studied. There do appear to be some interesting differences between countries, as well as between ethnic groups within a given country.

These diseases are much less common in Asia, but this may be changing. In Japan, for example, Crohn's disease was almost unheard of over half a century ago, but there appears to have been a steady increase in the incidence since then. The incidence in the Jewish population is among the highest of any ethnic or racial group. However, within the Jewish population, there appears to be a difference in incidence depending upon the country of origin. In one study, the incidence of IBD was higher in Jews of Ashkenazi (European) descent than in Jewish populations of Sephardic (Northern African and Middle Eastern) descent.

The varying risks of IBD in different countries are not entirely due to purely inherited or genetic reasons. The increasing incidence of Crohn's disease observed in Japan suggests that environmental factors have an important effect on the risk of developing IBD. In addition, studies of South Asian immigrants to North America have shown that the individuals who immigrate keep the lower risk of IBD that is seen in their country of origin, whereas their children, who are generally born and raised in North America, have a higher risk of developing IBD in their lifetime. These variations in the incidence of IBD provide clues as to the possible contributing factors or causes and have led to a number of interesting theories and questions that are undergoing further testing.

North-South Gradient

The incidence of IBD has generally been highest in North America and Northern European countries and lower in the countries at more southerly latitudes. This has been described as a "north-south gradient." However, this gradient is not unique to the north-south comparison but probably reflects an underlying gradient between developed and developing countries.

Where in the Body Does IBD Occur?

Inflammatory bowel disease occurs in specific sections of the gastrointestinal tract, or gut. Before considering what has gone wrong in Crohn's disease and ulcerative colitis, we need to understand how a healthy gut works. The normal functioning of the intestinal immune system may go awry in inflammatory bowel disease.

Functions of the Gastrointestinal Tract

The gastrointestinal tract is a tubular structure that extends from the mouth all the way down to the anus. The gut has two vital functions — nutrient absorption and immune protection.

Critical for Life

The gastrointestinal tract serves several critical functions that help to keep us alive. It allows nutrients, water, minerals, and vitamins to enter our body while keeping out harmful substances.

Principal Parts of the Gastrointestinal Tract

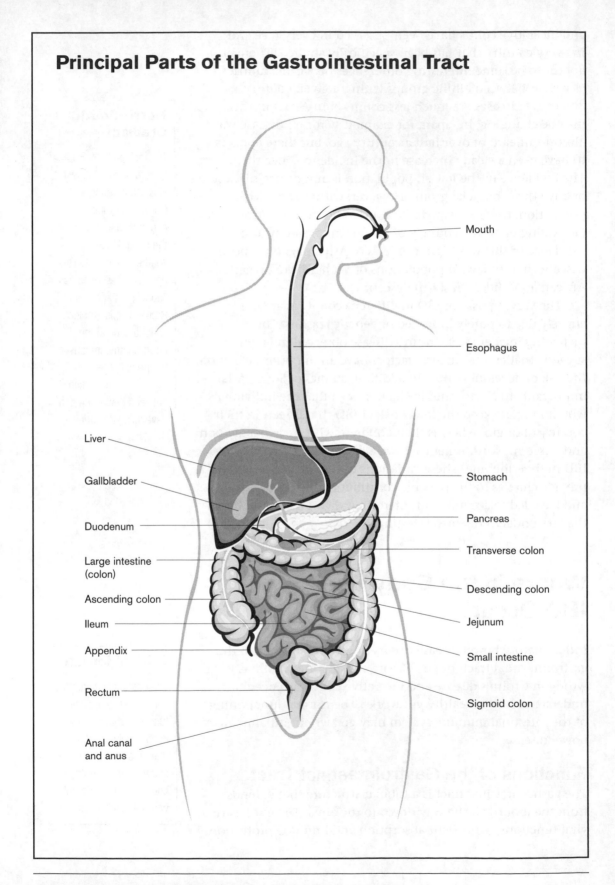

Mouth

Esophagus

Liver

Gallbladder

Duodenum

Large intestine (colon)

Ascending colon

Ileum

Appendix

Rectum

Anal canal and anus

Stomach

Pancreas

Transverse colon

Descending colon

Jejunum

Small intestine

Sigmoid colon

Nutrient Absorption

The primary job of the gut is to take in and absorb nutrients. These nutrients provide the building blocks and fuel needed to maintain all other bodily functions. The gut absorbs water, minerals, and vitamins from the food and drinks that are ingested.

Immune Protection

At the same time that it allows or promotes absorption of nutrients, the gastrointestinal tract must keep numerous potentially harmful items out of the body. These include microscopic organisms, such as bacteria, viruses, and parasites, as well as certain dangerous proteins that may cause disease if absorbed into the body from the gut. The gastrointestinal tract is, therefore, an important part of the body's immune system.

Principal Parts of the Gastrointestinal Tract

The gastrointestinal tract has six major components: mouth, esophagus, stomach, small intestine, large intestine, and anus. These may all be affected by inflammatory bowel disease.

Mouth

The mouth and the structures within it (lips, teeth, tongue, and palate) are involved in the ingestion of food. The teeth allow the grinding of food into small particles that are more easily broken down and digested by the enzymes present farther down in the intestine. The lips, tongue, and palate assist with the chewing and swallowing of food.

Esophagus

The esophagus (or gullet) is a tube that transports food, once it is swallowed, from the mouth to the stomach. A valve at the bottom of the esophagus prevents food and stomach acid from coming back up into the esophagus and into the mouth, where it can cause heartburn, which can result in damage to the inner lining of the esophagus. When you vomit, this valve opens up to allow acid and food to come out, and when you burp, it opens to allow gas to come out.

Stomach

This saclike structure lies in the upper part of the abdomen. It receives and holds food that has recently been eaten and slowly pushes it down into the small intestine, where most of the absorption of nutrients occurs. There is a valve at the lower end of the stomach that helps to regulate how quickly the food leaves the stomach to enter the small intestine. The stomach

IBD Ulcers

An area that has lost its mucosal lining is called an ulcer. When people talk about ulcers, they are usually referring to duodenal or gastric (stomach) ulcers, which are typically different from the ulcers that may occur in inflammatory bowel disease. In Crohn's disease and ulcerative colitis, the ulcers usually occur in the small intestine and large intestine and much less commonly in the stomach and duodenum.

provides an important signal to the brain to indicate when you have eaten enough.

The stomach also secretes acid from its lining. This helps to protect against infections caused by harmful bacteria that might inadvertently be ingested during a meal. The stomach acid also helps with the initial digestion of proteins in food. An enzyme called pepsin, also produced by the stomach, provides additional help with breaking down proteins.

Small Intestine

The small intestine (or small bowel) is a tubular structure approximately 12 to 15 feet (4 to 5 m) long. It is divided into three segments: from top to bottom, these are the duodenum, the jejunum, and the ileum. In the small intestine, most of the nutrients in food are absorbed into the body.

Mucosa

The absorption of nutrients is dependent upon the presence of a highly specialized inner lining (or mucosa). The mucosa lining is made up of cells whose main reason for being is to absorb nutrients from the inside (or lumen) of the intestine and pass them through into the body, where they are available as building blocks or fuel for other body functions. The surface of the mucosa is folded into many tiny fingerlike projections, called villi, which effectively increase the surface area and, therefore, the number of cells available for absorption of nutrients.

The surface of these cells contains enzymes that help break down food into smaller components so as to be absorbed more easily. When the intestine is inflamed, as is the case in inflammatory bowel disease, the villi may be reduced in number or size — or may be wiped out altogether so that the inner lining of the intestine appears flat. This loss of normal villi results in a reduced ability to absorb nutrients. When the inflammation is severe, the mucosa lining may be completely gone, leaving the underlying tissue exposed to the inside of the intestine.

Large Intestine

The large intestine, also known as the colon, is approximately 3 to 4 feet (1 to 1.2 m) in length. Although shorter than the small intestine, it is called the large intestine because its width or diameter is greater than that of the small intestine. It is divided into several sections: cecum, ascending colon, transverse colon, descending colon, sigmoid colon, and rectum.

Small Intestine

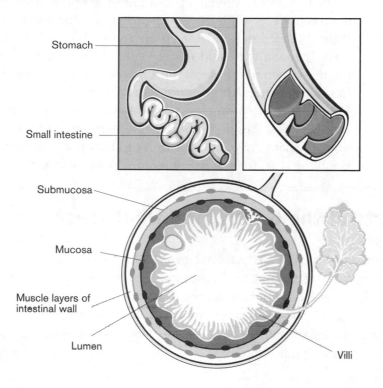

Stomach

Small intestine

Submucosa

Mucosa

Muscle layers of intestinal wall

Lumen

Villi

Large Intestine

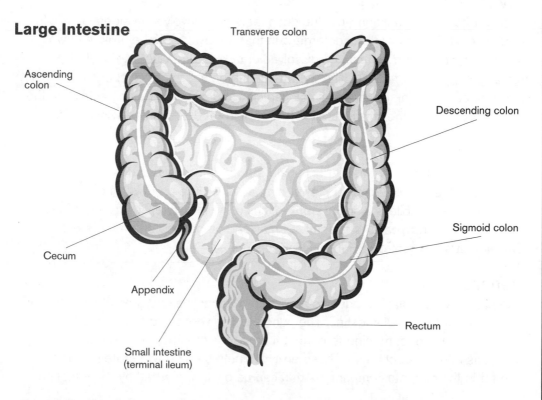

Transverse colon

Ascending colon

Descending colon

Cecum

Sigmoid colon

Appendix

Rectum

Small intestine (terminal ileum)

Rectum

The last part of the large intestine is called the rectum. The wall of the rectum can stretch, up to a certain point, to allow stool to be kept inside until there is an appropriate time to evacuate. When the rectum is inflamed or somehow diseased in other ways, that ability to hold stool is reduced, and you may feel the need to go to the bathroom very frequently and urgently. In some instances, this can result in accidents with associated loss of control of bowel function, otherwise known as fecal incontinence. This need for frequent bathroom visits and the urgency that may go along with it can be one of the most troubling symptoms of inflammatory bowel disease.

Related Parts of the Gastrointestinal Tract

There are other parts of the gastrointestinal tract involved to a greater or lesser extent in digestion and nutrient absorption. These organs, which are typically connected to the tubular part of the gastrointestinal tract by small channels (or ducts), include the liver, gallbladder, and pancreas. The gallbladder and pancreas are usually not affected by inflammatory bowel disease. However, the liver may be affected in a small proportion of patients. Occasionally, this can lead to liver damage.

Liver

The liver has many functions, but the one that is most involved in digestion is bile production. Bile is similar to a detergent, in that it allows fat to be broken down and made into a form that can be dissolved or mixed with water. Normally, fat remains separate from water, like the fat floating on the top of chicken soup. This ability of bile to break up fat into small particles and disperse those particles in the watery contents of the small intestine is crucial to fat digestion and absorption.

Gallbladder

Bile that is produced by the liver is usually stored in the gallbladder, a small sac next to the liver, until it is needed after a meal. When the production of bile is not adequate or if bile is blocked from reaching the intestine, absorption of fat from the diet is reduced. As a result, fat may end up coming out in the stool. This appears as droplets of fat or oil in the stool.

Pancreas

The pancreas is a gland producing a number of digestive enzymes that enter the upper part of the small intestine. The pancreas lies very close to the duodenum and has a small duct running through it that carries the enzymes from the pancreas into the duodenum. These enzymes help break down protein, starch, and fat in the diet into components that can be easily absorbed by the intestine.

Anus

The anus (or anal canal) is the passageway that stool follows when it leaves the body. The primary role of the anus is to keep the stool that is present in the rectum from coming out when you don't want it to come out. In other words, it helps to prevent fecal incontinence. Within the anal canal, there are two main muscular anal sphincters (or valves) that help to prevent the stool from coming out involuntarily.

One of the sphincters, called the external anal sphincter, is under your conscious control. In other words, you can control or tighten this particular sphincter when trying to hold in stool or gas. The other sphincter, the internal anal sphincter, is not under voluntary control, but works reflexively at a subconscious level. Maintaining continence and ensuring the smooth and complete emptying of the rectum requires the coordination of the two anal sphincters. If either of these two sphincters is damaged or diseased, it can result in fecal incontinence.

Signs of Inflammation

Inflammation occurs in response to any sort of injury, whether it is from a serious or life-threatening infection or from something as small as a paper cut. The classic signs of inflammation are pain, swelling, redness, and loss of normal function.

What Goes Wrong in IBD?

Crohn's disease and ulcerative colitis involve inflammation of the gut. A healthy person normally has a certain degree of inflammation in the gastrointestinal tract, but in those with IBD, the inflammation is extensive and excessive.

Normal Intestinal Inflammation

In the gut, the degree of inflammation that is normally present in healthy people is usually not enough to cause loss of function or to be seen by the naked eye, but when viewed under the magnification provided by a microscope, you can always see some white blood cells, called lymphocytes, present within the inner lining and just beneath the lining of the intestine.

These defensive cells are part of the intestine's immune system and help to protect you from potentially harmful bacteria, viruses, parasites, and proteins that aren't normally present in the body. The amount of inflammation is closely regulated so that there is just enough immune response so as to protect against these dangers, but not so much that it will cause problems.

Too much of a good thing may be bad, and the amount of inflammation in the intestinal lining is no exception. If there is too much inflammation or if it is not properly controlled, inflammation can cause swelling and damage to the tissues of the gastrointestinal tract. This damage can lead to problems

Excessive Inflammation

Excessive or uncontrolled inflammation is central to the onset of Crohn's disease and ulcerative colitis. As scientists learn more about the factors that control the degree of inflammation in the gut, they learn more about the causes of these disorders.

with the normal functioning of the gastrointestinal tract, including absorption of nutrients and fluids and retaining and expelling stool at appropriate times.

When the damage is particularly severe, the internal lining of the gastrointestinal tract can slough off, leading to a variety of symptoms, such as abdominal pain, diarrhea, blood in the stool, weight loss, and failure of children to grow properly.

Ulcerative Colitis Signs

Inflammation in ulcerative colitis is limited to the colon, but the extent of the inflammation within the colon varies from person to person and may vary within an individual over the course of the illness.

Any portion of the colon may be inflamed in ulcerative colitis, leaving the remainder completely unaffected. However, the rectum is always inflamed or diseased.

Pancolitis

In many instances, the entire colon is inflamed. This is referred to as pancolitis. When the inflammation extends upward, it does so in a continuous fashion. In other words, there are no areas of inflammation separated from one another by normal areas of colon.

Proctitis

In some people with ulcerative colitis, only the rectum is inflamed. This particular form of the disease is often referred to as proctitis or ulcerative proctitis. Some differences have been observed between proctitis and the more extensive forms of the disease, such as pancolitis. Ulcerative proctitis is unusual in children and tends to be seen more often when the disease occurs for the first time in middle-aged or elderly individuals.

Crohn's Disease Signs

In Crohn's disease, the inflammation can occur in any part of the gastrointestinal tract. Although it appears most often in the ileum and colon, Crohn's disease can affect the esophagus, stomach, duodenum, and jejunum.

Skip Lesions

The areas of the gut affected by Crohn's disease may not be adjacent to one another. These are called skip lesions. For example, someone with Crohn's disease may have an area of inflammation in the middle part of the small intestine (jejunum) and another area of inflammation in the large intestine, with normal intestine in between the two areas of inflammation.

Limited Extent

Because the extent of inflammation in ulcerative proctitis is so limited — involving at most just the last 6 inches (15 cm) of the large intestine — patients suffering from that form of the disease are usually not as sick as patients with more extensive forms of ulcerative colitis.

Intestinal Penetration

In ulcerative colitis, the inflammation tends to be limited to the innermost lining of the gut, but in Crohn's disease, the inflammation has a tendency to penetrate from the innermost lining, where inflammation and ulcers first occur, right through the deeper layers of the bowel to the outer surface (serosa). This results in a defect or hole in the bowel wall, which can lead to localized infections in the abdominal cavity (abscesses) or communications (fistulas) from the bowel into other organs or into the abdominal wall or skin. The inflammation in Crohn's disease may also form into tiny localized collections of inflammatory cells, called granulomas, which can be seen only under the magnification provided by a microscope. These granulomas are virtually diagnostic of Crohn's disease.

Site Variation

The wide variation in the sites of the gut that are affected by Crohn's disease can lead to important differences in the ways individual patients experience the disease and the ways in which they come to medical attention. This variation in sites also affects approaches to management of the disease.

Indeterminate Colitis Signs

In a small proportion of individuals with inflammatory bowel disease involving the colon, it is not possible, based on the disease features, to differentiate between ulcerative colitis and Crohn's disease. In these instances, the condition is designated as indeterminate colitis or inflammatory bowel disease of undetermined type (IBDU). In some cases of indeterminate colitis, the pattern of disease will change over time, and it will become apparent that the patient, in fact, has ulcerative colitis or Crohn's disease. However, some patients will continue to have features of both ulcerative colitis and Crohn's disease, and distinguishing between the two will not be possible.

The approach to the management of the two conditions with medications is similar. Differentiation becomes much more important if surgery is contemplated as a means of treatment, as the surgical approaches in ulcerative colitis and Crohn's disease can be quite different because of the fact that Crohn's disease can come back after surgery in parts of the bowel that weren't affected before surgery.

What Are the Possible Complications of IBD?

There are several serious complications that can occur as a result of having inflammatory bowel disease. This is where the danger lies. Some complications are common to Crohn's disease and ulcerative colitis, whereas others are unique to one form of IBD or the other. Generally, the complications can be divided into those that occur directly from the inflammation or ulceration that occurs in the intestine and those that occur in areas of the

Complications Specific to Crohn's Disease

- Strictures
- Abscesses
- Fistulas

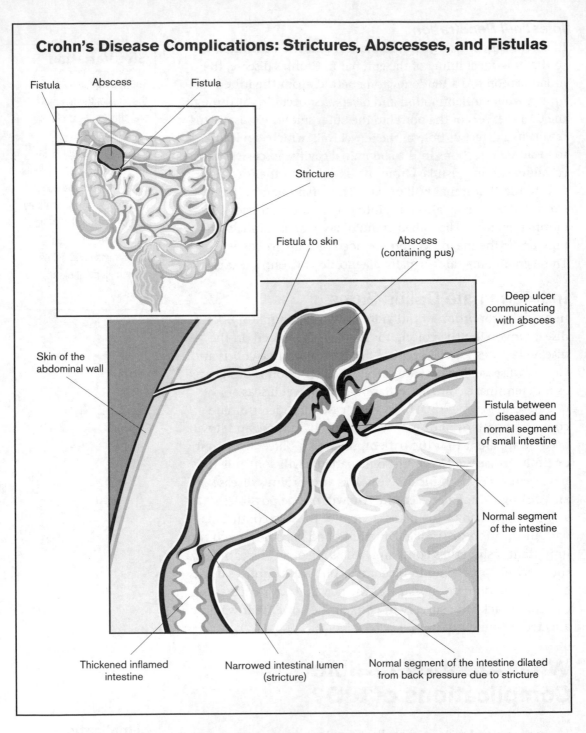

Crohn's Disease Complications: Strictures, Abscesses, and Fistulas

Fistula

Abscess

Fistula

Stricture

Fistula to skin

Abscess (containing pus)

Deep ulcer communicating with abscess

Skin of the abdominal wall

Fistula between diseased and normal segment of small intestine

Normal segment of the intestine

Thickened inflamed intestine

Narrowed intestinal lumen (stricture)

Normal segment of the intestine dilated from back pressure due to stricture

body that are not directly connected to the intestine or directly related to the intestinal inflammation.

Inflammation and Ulceration Complications

Inflammation and ulcerations can lead to strictures, fistulas, and abscesses in the gut. If these complications are not properly

What are strictures?

 Strictures are segments of the intestine in which the normally large internal opening becomes narrowed. This can be due to the swelling that occurs in the tissues of the intestinal wall as a result of active inflammation, similar to the swelling you get when you experience an injury, such as a broken bone. More often, the stricture is due to scarring of the intestinal tissues following repeated or ongoing episodes of inflammation and healing.

managed, they can, in turn, lead to further tissue damage and uncontrolled infection. Death can occur if this happens. While these complications are often seen in Crohn's disease, they are very rare in ulcerative colitis.

Strictures

Strictures are not necessarily a problem until they cause a bowel obstruction, commonly referred to as a blockage. Food or other material becomes caught in the narrowed stricture, preventing anything else from passing through. This produces back pressure in the intestine "upstream" from the stricture, causing sharp, often crampy pain, a distended abdomen, and nausea and vomiting. Sometimes there may be warning signs that a stricture may be worsening or leading to an obstruction. These signs include frequent or recurrent pain in the center of the abdomen after eating, along with a feeling of distension or bloating of the abdomen.

> **Foods to Avoid When You Have an Intestinal Stricture**
>
> - Popcorn
> - Nuts
> - Seeds
> - Corn
> - Raw vegetables
> - Skins on fruits

Bowel Obstruction

Not everyone with a stricture develops intestinal obstruction. If you experience a bowel obstruction that is not severe and know the symptoms, you can sometimes manage it on your own by avoiding solid food and drinking only fluids for several hours or even a few days. If you have a stricture, it is important that you avoid eating foods that aren't easily digested and that, as a result, may get lodged in the narrowed part of the intestine. These foods include popcorn, nuts, seeds, corn, raw vegetables (particularly stringy ones like celery), and skins on fruits.

This complication can be an emergency situation. You will usually require monitoring in a hospital setting, with intravenous fluids given to prevent dehydration and possibly the insertion of a nasogastric tube (a plastic tube inserted through the nose and down the esophagus into the stomach) to take fluid and gas out of the stomach.

Bowel Obstruction Symptoms

- Severe crampy pain, usually centered in the middle of the abdomen
- Distension or bloating of the abdomen
- Reduced number of bowel motions
- Not passing gas
- Nausea and vomiting

Not all symptoms are necessarily present when a bowel obstruction has occurred, particularly if it is partial or incomplete.

Immediate Medical Attention

If there is fever with the stricture symptoms, if there is frequent vomiting, or if after 6 to 8 hours symptoms of the obstruction are not starting to clear, as evidenced by reduced pain, decreased abdominal distension, and resumption of normal bowel motions and passing gas, then immediate medical attention is needed.

If the obstruction does not settle with these measures, then surgery is usually required to remove the strictured area of bowel. Fortunately, most obstructions that are due to Crohn's disease strictures settle without the immediate need for surgery, but repeated obstructions usually mean that surgery is required. In that instance, the surgery can be scheduled electively so that it is performed when you are well nourished, not sick, and not on medications that might affect healing and recovery after surgery. Medications are not very effective at relieving obstruction, particularly when the narrowing is due to scarring.

Abscesses

When a deep ulcer penetrates through all of the layers of the intestine, the contents of the intestine, primarily bacteria and fecal material, can leak out and into the abdominal cavity and tissues around the intestine. When a lot of this material leaks out suddenly, it can produce a serious, and occasionally fatal, infection called peritonitis.

In Crohn's disease, this leakage normally occurs very gradually, and the tissues around the intestine have a chance to react and to form a barrier against free leakage of the bacteria into the abdominal cavity. As a result, the bacteria accumulate in a localized area that is effectively walled off. The bacteria grow in the center of this walled-off region, causing a localized infection known as an abscess. An abscess typically contains pus in its center.

Serious Bacterial Infection

When an abscess is not properly treated, it can grow in size. Eventually, the bacteria can spread into the bloodstream and throughout the body, or it can burst into adjacent organs and tissues or into the abdominal cavity, causing the pus to spread throughout the abdomen. Any of these situations can be extremely serious or life threatening.

Fistulas

Fistulas are abnormal channels or tracts joining one part of the intestine to another part of the intestine or to another organ. When an area of the intestine becomes inflamed and ulcerated, the ulcer can penetrate through the full thickness of the intestine wall into an adjacent tissue. This is promoted by the fact that inflamed intestine tends to be "sticky" on its outside surface and will attach to other adjacent segments of intestine, to surrounding organs, or to the inner surface of the abdominal wall.

When a fistula forms between two segments of intestine, there may be no obvious bad consequences, but it is possible that the fistula can result in ingested food bypassing large segments of the intestine. This can cause decreased absorption of nutrients, leading to weight loss and malnutrition. Fistulas can pass from the intestines to adjacent organs, such as the bladder, which, in turn, leads to recurrent urinary infections.

Perianal Fistulas

The most common type of fistula occurs in the area around the anus. These anal fistulas are thought to arise from an infection or inflammation in the glands just below the lining of the anal opening. The infection or inflammation can burrow in various directions through the surrounding tissues and eventually open onto the skin in the area outside the anus. These types of fistulas, also called perianal fistulas or perineal fistulas, can be extremely distressing, and, for some individuals, dominate all other manifestations of their Crohn's disease.

People with perianal fistulas can have ongoing episodes of pain around the area of the anus, along with swelling and drainage of mucus, pus, blood, and stool. In women, the inflammation and fistulas can extend from the area around the anus to the area of the vagina. When they are particularly severe, the symptoms related to fistulas can interfere with everyday activities, such as sitting, walking, exercising, and riding a bike.

Pain and Shame

When a fistula goes from the intestine to the skin of the abdominal wall or around the anus, intestinal fluid or stool comes out through the opening of the fistula on the skin. In addition to being unsightly, this intestinal fluid makes it difficult to keep the area clean and can be irritating to the surrounding skin.

Because of the location of some fistulas, they can also get in the way of some types of sexual activity. This is not simply a result of the pain that may be associated with a fistula, but also of the potential embarrassment or shame of being "unclean." If you have these feelings, it is important to realize that you are not alone. Discussing your concerns with your partner will often help soothe some of your fears and concerns about being intimate. Together, you may even be able to come up with sexual activities or positions that you both find pleasurable and that you will not find painful or uncomfortable.

Extra-Intestinal Manifestations

Both Crohn's disease and ulcerative colitis may be associated with inflammation of tissues outside of the intestinal tract, specifically the joints, eyes, skin, and liver. The extra-intestinal manifestations often occur when the intestinal disease is more active or symptomatic, but they can also occur when the bowels are not giving any trouble at all. Unfortunately, there is no good way to predict who might get these particular complications, nor do we know how to prevent them from occurring. We do know that certain complications have some genetic or inherited basis contributing to their occurrence in IBD.

Joint Inflammation

Joint symptoms are probably the most common extra-intestinal manifestation of IBD, occurring in up to 30% of patients. The joints that are most commonly affected are the knees, ankles, wrists, and small joints in the fingers (knuckles) and toes. Symptoms of joint involvement or inflammation include pain and stiffness in the joints or, when severe, swelling and redness.

Sacroiliitis

A specific type of arthritis, called sacroiliitis, can occur in the lower back of patients in both Crohn's disease and ulcerative colitis. This typically presents first with stiffness in the lower back in the mornings and a vague discomfort over the lower back or hips. In a more severe form, called ankylosing spondylitis, the inflammation can extend up the spine, ultimately causing the bones of the spine to fuse together, thereby reducing flexibility and mobility. For ankylosing spondylitis, there is a blood test that can predict who is at risk for developing it, but unfortunately there is really no way to prevent its development.

Eye Inflammation

Eye inflammation is a relatively uncommon, but potentially serious, occurrence in IBD. There are several different, though closely related, forms of eye inflammation that can occur (called iritis, uveitis, and episcleritis), which all lead to red and often painful eyes. In some instances, the pain is made worse by bright lights, and there may also be blurring of vision. Any of these symptoms should be assessed promptly by a doctor and treatment started. The usual treatment is medicated eye drops containing steroids, but these should be used only after a proper examination by a qualified practitioner.

Complications of IBD Outside the Intestine (Extra-Intestinal Manifestations)

- Joint symptoms (pain, stiffness, swelling)
- Sacroiliitis
- Eye inflammation
- Skin lesions
- Liver disease (primary sclerosing cholangitis)
- Bone disease

Compounded Problems

Unfortunately, some of these joint problems, particularly sacroiliitis, tend to persist even when the underlying bowel disease is adequately treated and controlled. To compound the problem, some of the drugs commonly used to treat joint inflammation, such as nonsteroidal anti-inflammatory drugs, may be harmful to the intestinal tract of patients with IBD.

Skin Lesions

There are two main types of skin lesions that can be seen occasionally, but not frequently, in patients with IBD: erythema nodosum and pyoderma gangrenosum. Although it isn't known for certain if early treatment of the skin lesions of IBD result in better outcomes, it is important to be aware of any skin lesion that is particularly painful or enlarging for no apparent reason.

A third type of skin lesion, psoriasis, although not directly caused by IBD, can be seen more frequently in IBD, particularly in patients with Crohn's disease. Psoriasis typically results in red, raised, scaly, and itchy rashes that can occur just about anywhere on the body. What is interesting is that Crohn's disease and psoriasis share some genetic factors that increase the risk of both conditions, and the drug treatments of the two inflammatory conditions overlap. Some therapies, such as treatments based on the antitumor necrosis factor (infliximab or adalimumab) or on anti-interleukin-12/23 (ustekinumab), may be effective for both.

Erythema nodosum

The lesions of erythema nodosum are red or purplish, raised, and painful. They occur most often on the shins. They typically appear when the bowel symptoms are more active and go away as the bowel disease responds to treatment, sometimes leaving a small area of discoloration.

Pyoderma gangrenosum

Pyoderma gangrenosum is an area of ulcerated skin that usually occurs on the legs, but can occur on other areas of the body, particularly near the site of an ileostomy or colostomy. The lesion is sometimes painful, but it often looks much worse than it feels. The ulcerated area can grow to be quite large — sometimes 2 inches (5 cm) or even more across — and fluid can often ooze

---

Enlarging Lesions

- Patients often say that erythema nodosum and pyoderma gangrenosum lesions seem to start with what they thought was a bruise or an insect bite but quickly enlarge and worsen. When this happens, a doctor should be notified promptly.

- The drug infliximab has been shown to be particularly effective at healing pyoderma gangrenosum lesions.

Skin Rashes

Although treatments based on the antitumor necrosis factor (infliximab, adalimumab, and golimumab) may be effective at treating the skin lesions associated with IBD, their use may also result in unusual skin rashes. These are generally not serious and can usually be managed with creams or ointments applied to the site of the rash. In rare cases, these drugs can be associated with new onset of a skin condition called psoriasis or, in some cases, a worsening of psoriasis that was present prior to the start of therapy. This is an unusual reaction to therapy because these drugs are usually quite effective at treating psoriasis.

from its surface. Although it may improve when the bowel disease is treated, it does not always. When the lesions heal, they may leave areas of scarring or changed pigmentation.

Infliximab (Remicade) and adalimumab (Humira), two of the antitumor necrosis factor (anti-TNF) based treatments that are used to treat IBD, can be effective at healing pyoderma gangrenosum lesions.

Although it isn't known for certain whether earlier treatment of the skin lesions of IBD results in better outcomes with treatment, it is important to be aware of any skin lesion that is particularly painful, ulcerated, or enlarging for no apparent reason. Patients often say that erythema nodosum and pyoderma gangrenosum lesions seem to start off as what they thought was a bruise or an insect bite but quickly enlarge and worsen. When this happens, see your doctor promptly.

Liver

The most serious liver condition related to IBD is called primary sclerosing cholangitis (PSC). PSC appears to be somewhat more common in ulcerative colitis than in Crohn's disease, and when it occurs in Crohn's disease, there is often involvement of the large intestine (colon) with inflammation. PSC is thought to begin as an inflammation that specifically involves the small channels (ducts) carrying bile from the liver to the small intestine. It can lead to scarring and narrowing of these bile ducts, and, when severe or advanced, can result in damage to the liver. If the condition continues to progress, it can lead to liver cirrhosis and liver failure. PSC also predisposes the patient to episodes of bacterial infection of the bile ducts.

PSC is usually first suspected because of abnormal blood tests. This usually requires further tests or scans to see if the strictures characteristic of PSC are present. Occasionally, a liver biopsy may be necessary to sort out the possible causes. Most doctors will include blood tests of liver function and inflammation as a part of the routine checkup, even for individuals whose IBD is quite stable and not flaring. This may allow for earlier detection of PSC, but there is not an effective therapy that will prevent the progression of PSC to liver cirrhosis.

Mildly abnormal blood tests indicating liver inflammation or irritation are usually temporary and do not indicate any serious damage or long-term consequence to the liver. The abnormal blood tests are probably due to small areas of inflammation within the liver tissue that are a reaction to the associated bowel inflammation. It is not known how or why this occurs, but it tends to go away on its own and can recur repeatedly over time.

PSC Incidence

No more than 5% of people with IBD are affected by the serious liver complication called primary sclerosing cholangitis (PSC). If the condition continues to progress, it can lead to liver cirrhosis and liver failure.

Fever and Jaundice

In someone who has PSC, any episode of fever, particularly if it occurs with jaundice (yellow color) of the skin or eyes, needs to be assessed and treated immediately.

PSC is also associated with an increased risk of colorectal cancer. This increased risk requires specialized and intensive monitoring or surveillance with regular colonoscopies. PSC is also associated with an increased risk of bile duct cancer. Unfortunately, there is no good way to monitor for this complication.

Bone Disease

Although bone disease is not, strictly speaking, considered to be an extra-intestinal manifestation of IBD, individuals with IBD are at higher risk of developing certain types of bone disease. In the past, osteomalacia and rickets — serious problems with bone formation — were seen as a result of severe vitamin D deficiency in patients with Crohn's disease. These conditions are seldom seen now, probably as a result of better medical and nutritional treatments for patients with IBD.

Osteoporosis

Osteoporosis has been recognized as a prevalent condition. Osteoporosis involves a decrease in the density of the bone that occurs as a result of a reduction in the amount of minerals, such as calcium, in the bones. The bones are not strong and, therefore, susceptible to fracture with only minor trauma or sometimes without any apparent reason. Osteoporosis does not produce any symptoms until a fracture occurs.

While osteoporosis commonly occurs in older individuals without IBD, particularly in women, it seems to occur at an earlier age in patients with IBD. There are several reasons why IBD patients are more susceptible to developing osteoporosis at a younger age. The disease itself, particularly in Crohn's disease, and the associated inflammation appear to lead to reduced bone density, probably as a result of factors released into the bloodstream from the inflamed tissues. These factors, in turn, interfere with bone formation. Poor intake or absorption of certain key nutrients, such as calcium and vitamin D, may also play an important role in some patients. In addition, a person's overall nutritional state, as reflected by body weight, is also an important factor in determining bone density. In general, individuals who are underweight or malnourished tend to be more at risk of developing osteoporosis.

Medications

Medications are a major factor in the development of osteoporosis in IBD patients. In particular, steroid medications, such as prednisone, have been associated with an increased risk. Most doctors try to limit the duration of steroid treatment in

Minerals and Vitamins

For patients with IBD, maintaining an adequate intake of minerals and vitamins is an important means of preventing osteoporosis — not only good calcium and vitamin D intake but also good overall nutritional intake in terms of total calories and protein in the diet.

Osteoporosis Risk

People with IBD are at increased risk of developing osteoporosis, particularly if they have Crohn's disease or if they have received steroid medications. Some studies have indicated rates of osteoporosis of 30% in IBD patients. Osteoporosis appears to be more common in Crohn's disease than ulcerative colitis.

Most IBD patients, particularly those with Crohn's disease, should have their bone density measured and, if it is lower than normal, it should be checked periodically (every 1 to 2 years). Bone density is measured using a safe and easy test called a DEXA (dual energy X-ray absorptiometry), which doesn't require any injections.

their patients with IBD, and when starting someone on steroids, they will often recommend calcium and vitamin D supplements or start the patient on bisphosphonate medications (for example, etidronate, alendronate, zoledronate, and risedronate) that can help prevent further bone density loss. Most other medications used to treat IBD do not affect bone density.

The treatment of low bone density in children and adolescents with IBD is somewhat different than in adults. The period during adolescence and early adult life is critical in determining the health of the skeleton and bones in later life. People reach their maximum bone density in early adulthood. However, adolescents with IBD may not be able to reach their potential maximum bone density because of poor nutritional intake, because of the underlying IBD, or because of medications. Special attention needs to be paid to adequately treating the IBD, to maintaining good nutrition, and to minimizing use of steroids during these critical years.

Cancer

While people with IBD have an increased risk of cancer, this should not be a cause for undue concern.

Cancer is a common disease that can occur in many forms and degrees of seriousness. The increased risk of cancer in IBD patients appears to be limited to one or — at most — a handful of cancer types. Risk of colorectal cancer (cancer of the rectum or large intestine) appears to be most increased in individuals with IBD.

Some recent research has suggested that patients with more inflammation occurring over a period of many years are at increased risk, but colorectal cancers can also be found in people who have had a very mild IBD course.

While not everyone with IBD is at increased risk of developing colorectal cancer, it is important to be aware of the factors that do seem to increase the risk. For many years, only individuals with ulcerative colitis were considered to have an increased risk of colorectal cancer, but it now appears that people with Crohn's disease, where the large intestine is extensively affected, are also at increased risk. However, in those individuals with ulcerative colitis, where the disease is limited to the rectum and the last part of the colon, there is no significant increase in the risk of cancer. Patients diagnosed before 20 years of age, with more than an 8-year history of IBD or with associated primary sclerosing cholangitis, are at increased risk of colorectal cancer. The risk appears to increase further the longer one has had the disease. Patients with a family history of colorectal cancer involving a parent, brother, or sister are likely also at increased risk. Whether or not the severity of the IBD affects the cancer risk is not entirely known.

Risk Factors for Colorectal Cancer

- Extensive inflammation of the colon (ulcerative colitis or Crohn's colitis)
- Early age of diagnosis (less than 20 years of age)
- Long duration of disease (more than 8 years)
- Active disease symptoms
- Family history of colorec-tal cancer
- Primary sclerosing cholangitis (PSC)

Q **What can I do to reduce my risk of developing colorectal cancer now that I have IBD?**

A The first thing to do is to determine your degree of risk. This should be done in consultation with your doctor. If it is determined that you are at increased risk, by virtue of the risk factors, then it is possible that your doctor will recommend that you should enter into a screening program. Even if screening is not recommended, regular follow-up with your doctor is important.

You may have heard of colorectal cancer screening for individuals who do not have IBD. This is different from the screening that an IBD patient would require. Some of the methods of screening used for non-IBD individuals, such as testing the stool for microscopic traces of blood, are not effective for screening IBD patients. Monitoring for symptoms of cancer is not effective because the symptoms of colorectal cancer may be very similar to those of IBD. The screening that is carried out in IBD patients involves conducting a colonoscopy in order to take numerous random biopsy samples of the colonic lining. Although this type of screening program does appear to reduce cancer rates and result in cancers being detected earlier at curable stages, it is still not a perfect method.

In recent years, efforts have been made to detect precancerous changes by using newer colonoscopy technologies so that the areas of potential concern are made visible to the naked eye, allowing biopsies specifically targeted to those areas rather than the random biopsies that have been traditionally performed.

Dysplasia

Biopsies are carefully examined by a pathologist looking for precancerous changes, called dysplasia. If these changes are found, they indicate a higher possibility (10% to 20%) that the patient may already have cancer or, if cancer isn't already present, the patient has a substantial chance of developing cancer over the subsequent few years. When dysplasia is found and confirmed, surgery to remove the colon is usually recommended.

> ### Colorectal Cancer Risk
>
> It has been estimated that people with ulcerative colitis have a 10% to 15% risk of developing colorectal cancer during their lifetime.

Prevention and Treatment

Because we cannot yet predict with certainty who will suffer from inflammatory bowel disease and because the causes of this disease have not yet been determined conclusively, it is difficult to recommend effective prevention strategies. The best strategy for now is to learn how to recognize the symptoms of the disease and bring them to the attention of your doctor for immediate assessment, diagnosis, and treatment. In the next chapter, we present a discussion of the symptoms of inflammatory bowel disease and the tests used by doctors to diagnose this condition.

CHAPTER 2

How Do I Know I Have IBD?

CASE STUDY Jonathan

Jonathan is a 33-year-old police officer who has had several episodes of belly pain every 6 to 9 months during the past 5 years. Each time, these last between 2 and 6 weeks. Usually, the pain is crampy and tends to occur anywhere from 30 to 90 minutes after he eats. He feels bloated and uncomfortable. Jonathan also experiences watery diarrhea up to eight times a day during the pain episodes. The episodes subside on their own.

When the episodes occur, Jonathan's appetite is poor, and he can lose up to 10 pounds (5 kg). In between the episodes, he has no pain and regains most of the weight that he lost. However, during the past 2 years, he has felt more tired than usual.

Jonathan doesn't think much of these episodes. His wife has irritable bowel syndrome, a condition she has been told is related to diet and stress, and he figures that he has something similar. However, this year, Jonathan happens to have had his annual physical examination shortly after an episode of pain and diarrhea, and he mentions it in passing to his doctor.

After further questioning, his doctor is concerned that Jonathan may be suffering from something more serious than irritable bowel syndrome. He is concerned about the weight loss that occurs during the episodes and the fact that Jonathan wakes up from his sleep with pain and diarrhea. In addition, the doctor is able to feel a tender area of swelling in the lower right area of Jonathan's abdomen.

Based on these findings, the doctor is concerned that Jonathan may have Crohn's disease in the ileum (the last part of the small intestine). He decides to order tests to investigate further…

(continued on page 152)

Recognizing Symptoms

Sometimes, people, particularly young people, delay seeking medical attention for inflammatory bowel disease because they believe that they will remain healthy and that any symptoms they experience are likely due to simple conditions that are probably not long-lasting. Although some people feel that the symptoms are suspicious, they may deny the possibility of having a serious chronic disease, especially if they already have a family history of IBD and do not wish to face the possibility that they, too, are going to have to live with this disease. In some cases, the delay in diagnosis may be due to a general lack of knowledge on the part of the individual about what constitutes abnormal or unacceptable symptoms or due to embarrassment that they may feel in discussing their symptoms.

Another feature of IBD that may lead to a delay in diagnosis is the fact that the symptoms may come and go without any treatment, so that someone with IBD may have symptoms that go on for days or weeks and then go away on their own, and the person may feel perfectly healthy again for many weeks or months until the symptoms come back. With this pattern of symptoms, people may dismiss the episodes when they occur, thinking they will go away again on their own, and will often not mention them to their doctor or primary care provider.

Very occasionally, a delay in diagnosis may occur when a physician discounts a patient's description of symptoms or misses important clinical clues toward making the diagnosis.

For most people, any delay between the time symptoms begin and the time they ask their doctor for advice is due to the gradual change from a state of good health to a state of illness or disease. There are likely very few individuals with IBD who do not eventually undergo evaluation and have a diagnosis of Crohn's disease or ulcerative colitis confirmed.

Good Health
Crohn's disease and ulcerative colitis typically develop in people who previously were in good health and who had no prior bowel symptoms or digestive problems.

Common Symptoms

Inflammatory bowel disease — in particular, Crohn's disease — can present with quite different symptoms from one person to the next, and these symptoms depend upon many different factors.

Some factors are not directly related to the disease. These include usual bowel habits before developing IBD, pain tolerance or threshold, and probably even mood. Although these individual factors may modify the symptom experience, the nature of the inflammation — its severity, extent, and location — is most important in determining the symptoms.

Crohn's disease and ulcerative colitis tend to share a number of symptoms, such as abdominal pain and diarrhea, but they can be quite different with respect to the prominence of these symptoms and their course over time. The common symptoms of the two disorders and how they manifest are listed on the next page.

Flare Periods
Crohn's disease and ulcerative colitis fluctuate in severity, and patients can experience flares and remissions. Symptoms are typically experienced primarily during these flare periods. When the disease is in remission, patients, particularly patients with ulcerative colitis, may have no symptoms whatsoever.

Quick Guide to Ulcerative Colitis Symptoms

If you experience any one or combination of the following symptoms, be sure to consult with your doctor.

- Rectal bleeding (blood and mucus in the stool)
- Rectal urgency (frequent trips to the toilet and urgent need to move the bowels that often can't be delayed)
- Severe abdominal cramps
- Frequent diarrhea
- Increased intestinal gas
- Persistent fatigue
- Weight loss

Ulcerative Colitis Symptoms

Because ulcerative colitis affects only the large intestine, the symptoms are due to inflammation, damage, and ulceration of the lining of the large intestine. The inflammation is usually contained within the most superficial inner linings of the large intestine. This determines the type of symptoms that a patient may experience. Because of these symptoms, patients with ulcerative colitis often feel they have to stay close to a bathroom when their disease is active.

Rectal Bleeding

Blood in the stool occurs regardless of whether the inflammation is restricted to just the bottom end of the large intestine (rectum) or involves the entire large intestine. Mucus is often passed along with blood in the stool, but can sometimes occur on its own. In some cases, blood and mucus may be passed without any stool. Although this bleeding can happen with every bowel movement and can appear quite severe, it almost never results in a sudden fall in the hemoglobin (blood count), and, as a result, the bleeding is almost never an emergency situation. It is, however, an indication of the severity of the underlying inflammation and requires medical attention.

Other common conditions, such as hemorrhoids, can also cause blood with stools, so not all rectal bleeding is due to ulcerative colitis.

Blood in the Stool

The most obvious and consistent manifestation of ulcerative colitis is the presence of blood in the stool. This occurs in almost every individual with ulcerative colitis. In fact, if someone with IBD has never had blood in the stools, it is quite possible that the condition is Crohn's disease rather than ulcerative colitis. Crohn's disease is not always associated with blood in the stool.

Rectal Urgency

Inflammation of the rectum always occurs in ulcerative colitis and affects the normal ability to hold stool and gas. Patients with ulcerative colitis may experience frequent and very strong urges to move the bowels whenever there is the smallest amount of stool, blood, mucus, or gas in the rectum. This urgency is often accompanied by strong lower abdominal cramping that is probably due to contraction or spasm of the rectum and sigmoid colon.

When patients experience this type of urgency and are not close to a bathroom, they may not be able to control the urge long enough and may be incontinent. This loss of control can sometimes be the most troubling symptom for patients with ulcerative colitis. In many cases, individuals with active ulcerative colitis will plan their activities so that they always have easy and quick access to a bathroom.

The increased bowel activity usually occurs in the early-morning hours and soon after eating. As a result, patients will avoid going out in the morning until after bowel movements subside, or they will avoid eating before going out of the house. When the ulcerative colitis is more severe, the bowel activity may continue throughout the night and will make the patient wake up several times to go to the bathroom.

> **Unrelenting Pain**
>
> Between flares, patients usually do not feel any pain. If a patient with ulcerative colitis reports constant, unrelenting abdominal pain, it suggests the possibility of another diagnosis or a complication, such as bowel perforation. Be sure to consult with your doctor if abdominal pain has this characteristic.

False Urges

False urges are another troubling symptom that many patients with active ulcerative colitis experience. When the rectum becomes distended with gas or stool, it sends a signal to the brain indicating a need to move one's bowels. When the rectum is inflamed, it becomes irritable and will send these signals to the brain with only the smallest amount of distension or even without any distension at all.

In that case, a person will feel a strong urge to move the bowels and will rush to the bathroom, only to find that nothing comes out or, at most, just a small amount of blood and mucus. As a result, people with ulcerative colitis may have to make countless trips to the bathroom every day, even though they may pass stool only a handful of times.

Typically, when stool is passed, it comes in only small amounts each time. Because patients will pass what is recognized as stool only very infrequently, they will sometimes feel as if they are constipated. When only the rectum is inflamed, the inflammation and spasm may actually block the normal stool that is present in the large intestine above the rectum from getting through and being excreted.

Abdominal Pain

The inflammation of the inner lining of the intestine can produce abdominal pain, but because the inner lining of the intestine does not have nerve endings that can detect painful stimuli, abdominal pain is not a constant feature in most cases of ulcerative colitis. When it does occur, pain tends to be crampy, occurring around the time of bowel movements, and is often associated with rectal urgency. This pain is probably due more to the contraction or spasm of the intestine than to the inflammation of the inner lining itself.

Diarrhea

When the inflammation of the large intestine extends above the rectum, it affects the normal fluid-absorptive function of the large intestine, resulting in loose or liquid stools, also known as diarrhea. The liquid stool may be mixed with variable amounts of blood and mucus.

Intestinal Gas

Some patients experiencing a flare of ulcerative colitis will feel that they have an increased amount of gas or that the odor of the gas changes. Some even say that they can tell when a flare is about to come on because of this change in the odor. The amount of gas produced during a flare of colitis has never actually been studied, but it is likely that, even if the amount of gas produced is not increased, the inflamed rectum and large intestine are more sensitive to the presence of gas and, therefore, will pass it more frequently.

Fatigue

When the inflammation in the colon is particularly bad or when it involves a large portion of the colon, patients with ulcerative colitis may suffer from fatigue and weight loss. The fatigue is most often due to the inflammation itself, but can also be due to anemia resulting from blood loss in the stool. Chronic blood loss can, over time, lead to iron-deficiency anemia. When a person is anemic, the blood is not able to carry oxygen to the tissues in the body as effectively, and, as a result, a person may experience fatigue and breathlessness with minimal amounts of exertion.

Weight Loss

Cytokines can also produce changes in metabolism that result in loss of body weight, even when food intake is at a level that should be sufficient to maintain a person's healthy nutritional state.

Cytokines

Intestinal inflammation itself, even without producing anemia or iron deficiency, can also produce fatigue. This probably occurs as a result of certain proteins, called cytokines, that are released from inflamed tissues and that can produce symptoms such as fatigue, loss of appetite, and fever.

Crohn's Disease Symptoms

Crohn's disease can affect any part of the gastrointestinal tract. As a result, the symptoms reported by patients with Crohn's disease can be much more varied than those reported by patients with ulcerative colitis.

As with ulcerative colitis, the symptoms experienced in Crohn's disease are highly dependent upon the location and severity of the inflammation within the gastrointestinal tract. However, the relative prominence of the symptoms may be different in Crohn's disease than in ulcerative colitis. Because there are locations that are much more commonly affected than others, there are presenting symptoms that also tend to be more common than others. As a general rule, abdominal pain, diarrhea, fatigue, and weight loss tend to be the most common presenting symptoms in Crohn's disease. In children, failure to grow normally, or "failure to thrive," is a common presenting symptom.

Atypical Symptoms

Because the locations within the gut that are affected by the disease vary from person to person, there is no "typical" patient or "typical" symptom presentation in Crohn's disease.

Quick Guide to Crohn's Disease Symptoms

The symptoms of Crohn's disease are similar to the symptoms of ulcerative colitis. However, a number of additional symptoms, not typically experienced in ulcerative colitis, may be experienced in patients with Crohn's disease. One problem that is very uncommon in ulcerative colitis, but may be seen in Crohn's disease, is the occurrence of fistulas and abscesses around the anus and ulcers within the anal canal. These complications occur because of the tendency of Crohn's disease to penetrate more deeply into the bowel lining.

If you experience any one or combination of the following symptoms, be sure to consult with your doctor.

- Rectal bleeding (blood and mucus in the stool)
- Rectal urgency (frequent trips to the toilet and urgent need to move the bowels that often can't be delayed)
- Severe abdominal cramps
- Frequent diarrhea
- Increased intestinal gas
- Persistent fatigue
- Weight loss
- Fistulas and abscesses around the anus and ulcers within the anal canal
- Failure to grow or thrive in children

Tips for Working with Your Doctor

Working with your doctor to diagnose your symptoms is the first step in understanding and treating inflammatory bowel disease. However, some patients find their initial meeting with their doctor somewhat unsatisfactory because they do not have enough time to ask all the questions they may have. While most doctors do have busy schedules, you can make the most of your appointments with them by being well prepared. To get the most out of your visit to your doctor, try the following tips:

Make sure there is enough time.

If you think that your problems and concerns are going to take longer than the time your doctor usually allocates for an appointment, ask for a longer meeting. You will find this much more satisfactory than trying to "find a moment" at the end of the appointment to raise what may be your most pressing questions and concerns. If you do come to the end of your allotted time, acknowledge to the doctor that you have run out of time and that you still have items to discuss. The doctor may sometimes ask you to continue or, in some cases, suggest that you schedule another appointment.

Keep your description of symptoms focused and factual.

The doctor wants to hear about what you are feeling, so just describe what you are experiencing without jumping to conclusions or making speculations. You might say to your doctor, "I'm here today because I keep getting episodes when I can't move my bowels, my belly becomes distended like I'm 9 months pregnant, and I start vomiting. It feels exactly like it did when I had surgery for a bowel obstruction 4 years ago, but maybe a little less severe." Although you may suspect this is caused by a bowel obstruction, you don't need to interpret the experience or make a diagnosis. That is the doctor's job — to determine if the symptoms are due to a bowel obstruction or due to some other cause or condition that could produce similar symptoms.

Bring a list of your medications and their doses.

The doctor will need to know if you are taking any medications and their dosage. Report if you have experienced any side effects and when they first started in relation to when you began taking the medications.

Make a list of your questions and issues.

Keep your list of questions short enough that it can be covered in the available time and try to make sure that the questions are specific and to the point rather than being overly general and difficult to answer concisely. For example, answering a question such as "What are the possible side effects of this medication?" may take up the entire appointment, whereas asking "What are the common and serious side effects of this drug?" will get the information you are really looking for in a relatively short time, allowing time for other questions.

Prioritize your list of questions from most important to the least important.

Take care of the questions that are causing you the most concern first so that you can feel more at ease and more comfortable asking other questions. Often your doctor's answer to the most pressing question also answers other questions on your list.

Bring a friend or relative to help you remember what you have discussed.

Many patients ask a spouse, relative, or friend to accompany them to the appointment, to help them remember the questions they planned to ask and make note of the answers given by the doctor. Their emotional support is also important.

Make notes about key points in the discussion.

You or your companion should make a record of what your doctor investigates and concludes so that you can follow any treatment program the doctor may prescribe. This is especially important if treatment options are presented to you for your decision. You may want to refer to your notes when making your decision.

Q What is an abscess?

A The inflamed areas of the intestine may be tender to touch, so that any pressure applied to the abdomen may produce pain. When ulcers extend right through the intestinal wall, it can produce a reaction around the intestine, resulting in a swelling that can be felt by a physician examining the patient. Occasionally, this area can become infected by the bacteria from the intestine that are able to penetrate through the ulcer into the area of swelling. This is called an abscess. When this occurs, patients usually feel a constant pain over the affected area and may also have a fever.

Abdominal Pain

Unlike ulcerative colitis, where the inflammation is limited to the innermost lining of the intestine, in Crohn's disease, the inflammation and ulcers can penetrate through all the layers of the intestinal wall. Since there are nerves that can transmit pain signals in the deeper layers of the intestine, this means that pain may be a more consistent feature of Crohn's disease.

Strictures and Blockages

If Crohn's disease produces some narrowing of the intestine (most often in the small intestine), it can produce some degree of blockage, making it difficult for food and intestinal contents to get through the narrowed areas. This can be experienced as crampy abdominal pain that occurs within minutes to several hours after a meal, depending on the precise location of the narrowing. Bloating of the abdomen can occur along with this pain, and, when it is particularly severe, nausea and vomiting may also occur. More complete blockages can occur, and these will be associated with symptoms of abdominal pain, distension, nausea, and vomiting. During the episode, the person may not be able to pass any stool or gas.

Bowel Movements

As is the case in ulcerative colitis, patients with Crohn's disease may have crampy abdominal pain around the time of bowel movements. This may be due to irritability of the intestine and the associated spasm that can occur as a result of inflammation.

Immediate Medical Attention

Episodes of abdominal pain that last more than 4 to 6 hours without passage of gas or stool require immediate medical attention and often require hospitalization.

Diarrhea

Diarrhea is a common, but not universal, symptom of Crohn's disease. In fact, some patients with intestinal narrowing actually present with decreased bowel movements and constipation. The diarrhea that occurs in patients with Crohn's disease is usually not bloody, but when the lower part of the large intestine is inflamed, bleeding can occur more often.

Fatigue

Fatigue is a very common symptom in Crohn's disease and can be one of the most difficult symptoms to completely reverse with medical therapy. As in ulcerative colitis, it is probably due to the release of cytokines from the inflamed intestinal tissues.

Weight Loss

Weight loss may be due to the changes in metabolism caused by the cytokines, but it can also be caused by reduced nutrient intake as a result of pain that occurs after eating. In patients with small intestinal inflammation, there may be problems with absorption of nutrients, which can lead to weight loss.

Anal Problems

While patients with ulcerative colitis may describe irritation of the skin around the anus or may even develop hemorrhoids (swollen veins) because of the frequent bowel movements, patients with Crohn's disease are at risk of developing certain specific problems that are more serious. They can develop anal fissures or ulcers (painful breaks in the skin inside the anus), abscesses (painful collections of pus), and fistulas (small openings to the skin around the anus that can drain stool, pus, or blood).

Extra-Intestinal Symptoms

Both ulcerative colitis and Crohn's disease can present with certain associated symptoms or conditions outside of the intestine. These are called extra-intestinal manifestations and are usually due to inflammation of other tissues outside of the bowel — joints, eyes, skin, and liver, for example. Joint manifestations (arthritis) are the most common. These extra-intestinal manifestations can occur at the time of first diagnosis of IBD, or they can occur later on in the course of the disease. In occasional cases, they can first occur months or even years before the bowel symptoms first become apparent. The same major extra-intestinal manifestations and symptoms (joint, eye, skin, and liver) can occur in both disorders.

Nutrient Deficiencies

Depending on the part of the intestine involved in Crohn's disease, patients can develop specific nutrient deficiencies. For example, the last part of the small intestine (terminal ileum) is commonly affected in Crohn's disease; this is also where vitamin B_{12} is absorbed. As a result, vitamin B_{12} deficiency can develop in patients with Crohn's disease of the terminal ileum.

Onset of Symptoms

Inflammatory bowel disease usually first develops in one of three different patterns of symptom onset: gradual, sudden, and relapsing or remitting.

Gradual Onset

Most often, Crohn's disease and ulcerative colitis develop very gradually so that it takes many weeks, months, or, in some cases, years before patients recognize the symptoms and mention them to their doctor for diagnosis.

Sudden Onset

Unusually, though certainly not rarely, inflammatory bowel disease develops abruptly. Symptoms may come on suddenly, sometimes so quickly that the disease seems to develop virtually overnight, with the person going from a state of good health to a serious and severe illness without any obvious warning. This type of presentation is quite striking and can often make it very difficult for patients and their families. Important medical management decisions, including the choice of medications and the possibility of undergoing surgery, may be required before the patient has the chance to learn about the disease and its consequences, complications, and potential treatments.

Relapsing or Remitting Onset

Inflammatory bowel disease may also develop following a so-called relapsing or remitting course. Patients can present with mild episodes or flares that occur for days, weeks, or even months at a time. During these flares, symptoms get noticeably worse, but then seem to go away spontaneously (also called going into remission) so that the person goes back to a state of normal health with no symptoms for many weeks, months, or even years before another episode or flare occurs.

Because these flares often subside on their own, patients will sometimes not go to the doctor for investigation or treatment, until an episode is more severe, lasts longer than usual, or is more concerning in some way.

Diagnostic Methods

If you suspect you or a family member is experiencing any symptoms of inflammatory bowel disease, be sure to see your doctor as soon as possible. A medical history of symptoms and a physical examination are usually adequate for strongly

---

Diagnostic Tests for IBD

- Blood tests
- Stool tests
- Imaging studies
  - X-ray
  - Ultrasound
  - CT scan
  - MRI
- Endoscopy
  - Gastroscopy
  - Colonoscopy
  - Wireless capsule endoscopy
  - Enteroscopy
- Biopsies

---

suspecting a diagnosis of Crohn's disease or ulcerative colitis, but further diagnostic testing is important in confirming the suspected diagnosis, determining the extent and severity of the disease, and screening for possible complications of the disease. These procedures include standard blood and stool tests, various imaging studies, endoscopies, and biopsy.

Not all tests or investigations are required in all patients. The tests chosen will depend on your specific symptoms, as well as the availability, potential risk, and discomfort of the specific investigation.

Blood Tests

White blood cell or platelet count can increase in infections and inflammatory conditions and can be elevated in active IBD. Certain antibodies are found more frequently in the blood of patients with IBD. Antibodies are proteins produced by the immune system to defend against certain types of infection by binding to specific molecules found on the surface of viruses and bacteria. Some proteins, most commonly C-reactive protein, are found in higher levels in the blood of people with inflammatory conditions.

Antibody Patterns

The pattern of antibodies may help differentiate between ulcerative colitis and Crohn's disease. The antibodies found in the blood in IBD include anti-ompC, anti-CBir1, and anti-fla-X, among others. These are antibodies that target certain proteins found on bacteria. They have been combined in a commercially available blood test panel with some other proteins and genetic markers found in blood; together, these markers provide a probability of a given individual having IBD. One of these antibodies, called perinuclear antineutrophil cytoplasmic antibody (pANCA), occurs more commonly in ulcerative colitis, whereas another antibody, anti-Saccharomyces cerevisiae antibody (ASCA), is fairly specific for Crohn's disease.

There are several other antibody tests that are commercially available along with pANCA and ASCA. Although this panel of antibody tests cannot replace more definitive diagnostic tests, such as imaging studies, endoscopy, or biopsy, and although they cannot yet be used to confirm a diagnosis of IBD, they may be helpful in screening out patients with possible IBD before proceeding to more definitive and often invasive diagnostic testing. This may be particularly helpful in children, where invasive diagnostic testing is more difficult to justify and carry out, particularly when the suspicion of actually finding disease is relatively low. These antibody tests can be

> **Screening**
>
> Although blood tests cannot replace more definitive diagnostic tests, such as imaging studies, endoscopy, or biopsy, and although they cannot yet be used to confirm a diagnosis, they may be helpful in screening out patients with possible IBD before proceeding to more definitive and often invasive diagnostic testing.

used to help determine who should undergo further testing, since it is very unlikely that a child with a negative pANCA and ASCA test will turn out to have IBD. It also appears that, in a patient with known Crohn's disease or ulcerative colitis, certain patterns of the different antibodies, and the levels of antibodies present in the blood, may be associated with certain disease locations and with higher risk of developing certain complications of disease.

Other blood tests indicate evidence of possible complications or nutritional deficiencies that may have occurred as a result of IBD. These include blood tests for anemia, liver disease, iron deficiency, vitamin B_{12} deficiency, and calcium deficiency.

Stool Tests

Stool samples may be sent for culture to rule out a bacterial infection as the cause for a patient's symptoms. While the yield from this is quite low, particularly when symptoms have been going on for many weeks or even months, it is important to rule out infections before embarking on many types of therapy for Crohn's disease and ulcerative colitis.

Stool may also be examined for parasites or the eggs of parasites. Occasionally, the laboratory will report that no parasites were seen, but that many white blood cells are present in the stool. The presence of white blood cells almost always indicates some type of inflammatory condition in the intestine. Stool can also be tested for certain proteins — calprotectin and lactoferrin — that are present in white blood cells that indicate

Disease Activity

Stool tests can be used to monitor disease activity and response to treatment. These tests, when combined with blood tests, help make decisions regarding changes in treatment strategies.

the presence of active intestinal inflammation. The calprotectin level in stool has proven to be quite useful in people who present with symptoms that are not clearly or highly likely to be due to IBD. In that situation, an elevated calprotectin level is very suggestive of an underlying inflammatory condition such as IBD, and would support going ahead with other testing, such as endoscopy and biopsy, that can confirm the diagnosis.

X-Rays

Since the intestine does not appear in sufficient detail on plain X-rays, a contrast agent, usually barium, is used to fill the intestine so that the intestinal lining and wall can be seen in contrast to the barium. The barium is administered in several ways, depending on the area of bowel under examination. Because of the two-dimensional limitation of these techniques, they have been largely replaced by cross-sectional imaging studies, such as ultrasound, CT scan, and MRI.

Upper GI Series and Small Bowel Follow-Through

When examining the small intestine, the barium can be given by having the person drink it. X-rays are taken every few minutes as the barium passes out of the stomach and through the small intestine. This type of X-ray can also detect problems in the esophagus, stomach, and duodenum. It requires no preparation on the part of the patient other than having to fast on the day of the examination.

Small-Bowel Enema, or Enteroclysis

In some cases, a small-bowel follow-through X-ray doesn't provide enough detail because of problems with the movement of barium through the small intestine or because the images are captured only every few minutes and important information can be missed. To solve this problem, the barium is administered directly into the small intestine by means of a tube placed through the nose into the esophagus, stomach, and duodenum. The radiologist can watch continuously as the barium flows through the entire small intestine. This examination also requires only fasting prior to the procedure.

Barium Enema

Barium enema provides images of the large intestine (colon). Liquid barium solution and air are pumped into the large intestine. A barium enema is rarely performed, however, having been replaced by colonoscopy and CT scan.

X-Ray Risk

All X-rays involve some degree of exposure to radiation, but, as long as the tests are not repeated frequently, the amount of radiation exposure is relatively small compared to the amount that one is exposed to every day from background sources.

Conversely, a normal calprotectin level makes the likelihood of IBD much lower, and the doctor and patient or family may then decide against further testing. This decision can be of value when it comes to children, for whom a test such as endoscopy is more difficult to do.

Imaging Studies

Imaging studies provide "pictures" of the intestines and other internal organs without having to open up the abdomen by performing surgery. Imaging studies have been the mainstay of IBD diagnosis for many years. X-rays provide two-dimensional pictures of the intestine, while other types of imaging studies also provide information about surrounding structures within the abdomen, something which conventional X-ray studies cannot do. These include ultrasounds, computer-assisted tomography (CT, or CAT) scans, and magnetic resonance imaging (MRI). They provide multiple images of the abdomen in "slices" that can be positioned crosswise or lengthwise through the abdomen. In this way, it is possible to provide a three-dimensional representation of the intestines, other abdominal organs, and even blood vessels. Because of this capability, these imaging studies can provide improved diagnostic information compared with conventional X-ray studies.

Ultrasound

Ultrasound examinations are very safe and widely available. A probe that transmits a high-frequency sound wave is moved over the abdominal wall. That sound wave is reflected off structures within the abdomen and back to the probe, which has a sensor to detect the reflected sound waves, or echoes. These echoes are then converted into an image. Patients must fast before an abdominal ultrasound study. There are certain modifications of the ultrasound technique that can allow the radiologist to determine the rate of blood flow within the intestine. An increased blood flow may give an indication that the bowel is inflamed.

One particular type of ultrasound, a transanal ultrasound, is used to evaluate patients for possible anal abscesses and fistulas. This involves putting a special ultrasound probe into the anus in order to obtain images of the surrounding tissues. Although this may provide excellent detail, the procedure may be very difficult or impossible for patients with painful anal conditions associated with Crohn's disease.

Detecting Complications

Ultrasound may be helpful in detecting complications of IBD, such as abscesses, but it is not the most sensitive imaging study, particularly when the intestines are to be evaluated.

Computer-Assisted Tomography (CAT scan, or CT scan)

Computer-assisted tomography is a very safe and widely used imaging technique. This technology, along with MRI, has virtually replaced the small bowel follow-through and small-bowel enema procedures.

During a CT scan, the patient lies on a table, which is surrounded by a large donut-shaped structure that produces and detects X-rays. These X-rays are converted into very detailed images when processed in the machine's computer.

Patients undergoing CT scans of the abdomen are often given a contrast solution to drink 1 to 2 hours before the scan to provide better diagnostic images or an intravenous injection of another contrast material to show blood supply to the intestine and other tissues.

CT scans are generally not needed for routine follow-up of a patient's clinical disease activity. If an abscess is detected by CT scan, the images can be used by the radiologist to insert a needle or plastic tube through the skin and into the abscess in order to allow it to drain properly.

CT scans involve radiation exposure, which is always a concern, particularly in young people. However, newer "low-dose" CT scans expose patients to a fraction of the radiation that they would be exposed to with a standard CT scan, without losing much of the important diagnostic information.

Magnetic Resonance Imaging (MRI)

Magnetic resonance imaging is relatively new in IBD diagnosis. It uses a large magnet to create images based on the different water content and molecular makeup of different tissues. A patient undergoing an MRI scan lies on a table that slides into the machine. The patient lies very still during the procedure, which can last up to 20 or 30 minutes. Like a CT scan, the MRI provides cross-sectional images, but because the intestines are continuously contracting in the abdomen during the procedure, the images of the intestines may not be as clear as they are in CT scans, where the image is obtained in a fraction of a second. Some studies are done after patients are administered an injection of a contrast agent into the vein. Because it does not involve any exposure to radiation, MRI may become the investigation of choice once the technology has advanced to the point where it provides images that are comparable in quality to CT scans.

Sensitive Test

CT scans are very sensitive at detecting IBD complications, such as abscesses and intestinal obstructions. They do involve some radiation exposure and so should not be repeated too frequently or unnecessarily.

Assessing the Anus

MRI is particularly useful for assessing the anus and the surrounding tissue for complications, such as fistulas and abscesses, in Crohn's disease.

MRI is particularly useful for assessing the anus and the surrounding tissue for complications, such as fistulas and abscesses, in Crohn's disease. MRI is also useful in determining whether areas of the intestine are inflamed or whether the changes seen are due to scarring. This is a particularly helpful distinction because tissue that is inflamed may respond to therapy with medication, whereas areas of scarring will likely not improve with medical therapy.

Endoscopy

In endoscopy, a long, narrow tube with a light and a camera on its tip is passed into the gastrointestinal tract. The endoscope can be steered in the desired direction to provide very detailed images of the inner lining of the gastrointestinal tract on a video monitor. When the procedure examines the esophagus, stomach, and duodenum, it is called an upper gastrointestinal endoscopy or, more commonly, a gastroscopy. When the instrument is inserted through the anus into the rectum and colon, it is called a colonoscopy. When doing a colonoscopy, the physician can often also examine the ileum (last part of the small intestine). This is one of the areas most commonly involved in Crohn's disease.

Gastroscopy

Gastroscopy is a relatively straightforward procedure, but is done much less commonly in IBD than is colonoscopy, with the possible exception of individuals first diagnosed in childhood. In that case, gastroscopy is frequently carried out at the time of diagnosis. Gastroscopy is usually carried out following an overnight fast so that the stomach is empty. The back of the throat is sprayed with a local anesthetic so that the gag reflex is reduced, and, in some cases, a mild sedative is given intravenously to relax the patient. The whole procedure usually takes no more than 10 to 15 minutes and is typically not painful. In young children, it may be necessary to administer heavier sedation or general anesthetic in order to carry out the procedure.

Colonoscopy

Colonoscopy requires preparation of the bowel with a special diet (usually clear liquids) and a special laxative for one or more days prior to the procedure. This is important because the presence of feces can interfere with visibility and make the procedure almost useless. In some cases, the physician may not order a special laxative for the patient. Usually this is when the IBD is very active, but even in these instances, a smaller or more gentle preparation is probably still advisable and safe.

Upper Gastrointestinal Endoscopy

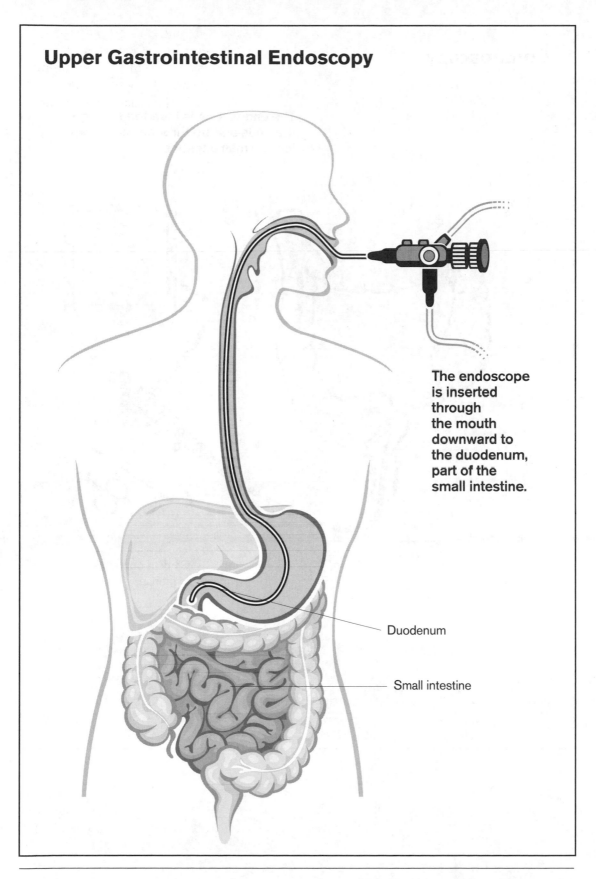

The endoscope is inserted through the mouth downward to the duodenum, part of the small intestine.

Duodenum

Small intestine

Colonoscopy

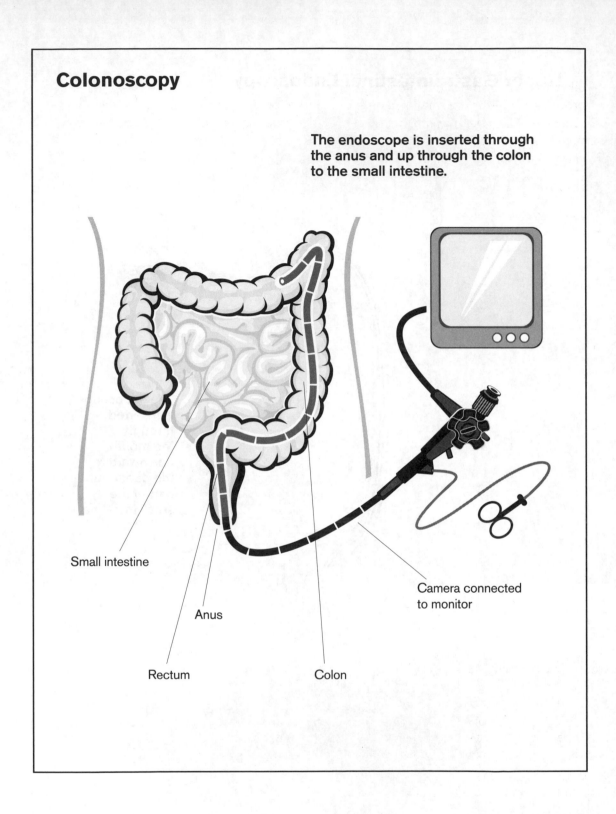

The endoscope is inserted through the anus and up through the colon to the small intestine.

Small intestine

Anus

Rectum

Colon

Camera connected to monitor

The colonoscopy procedure itself is usually performed with a sedative and an analgesic (pain medication). It typically takes 15 to 45 minutes to complete. It is generally quite a safe procedure, with a very small risk of serious complications, but some degree of abdominal pain and cramping is not unusual at times during the procedure. In most cases, the medication given before the procedure helps to minimize the discomfort.

Wireless Capsule Endoscopy

Standard gastroscopy and colonoscopy are not able to reach large segments of the small intestine that may be affected in Crohn's disease. The imaging studies that can take pictures of those areas of the small intestine are improving, but do not always provide the detailed images required by the physician to make management recommendations. Wireless capsule endoscopy (WCE), or PillCam technology, was developed to provide the types of high-quality visual images of the inner lining of the small intestine that are provided by gastroscopy in the stomach and duodenum and by colonoscopy in the colon and ileum. In most cases, the procedure allows examination of the entire length of small intestine.

A capsule — about the size of a large vitamin pill or capsule — that contains a battery, light source, and a tiny lens and camera chip is swallowed by the patient and begins taking two pictures every second during an 8-hour period. It is propelled through the esophagus, stomach, and small bowel by the normal muscular movements of the gastrointestinal tract in the same way food is passed down along the gastrointestinal tract. The patient wears a recording device, much like a cellular telephone, and can go about daily activities. Once the procedure is over, images are downloaded from the recorder to a computer. The physician can then look for signs of Crohn's disease.

Despite the fact that the WCE can provide excellent images of the entire small intestine, it is not commonly used in IBD diagnosis. In ulcerative colitis, the small intestine is not involved and does not require this type of detailed evaluation. In Crohn's disease, care must be taken because the capsule could produce a blockage or bowel obstruction in any strictures of the intestine. Nevertheless, the capsule may be helpful in diagnosing subtle degrees of Crohn's disease in the small intestine, where the other imaging techniques do not provide a full answer to the patient's symptoms.

> **Extremely Useful**
>
> Colonoscopy is an extremely useful diagnostic test in IBD. It will always detect ulcerative colitis if it is present, and will detect Crohn's disease in 80% to 90% of cases. In 10% to 20% of cases of Crohn's disease, the procedure is not able to examine the areas of disease because of technical factors or because the disease is beyond the reach of the colonoscope.

Enteroscopy

A number of innovations have been developed in the area of endoscopy to allow examination of areas of the small intestine that are beyond the reach of the standard gastroscope and colonoscope.

- Push enteroscopy uses a longer-than-normal gastroscope to get farther into the small intestine, but the success of this procedure is limited because of the floppiness and many twists and turns of the small intestine.

- Double balloon enteroscopy (DBE) generally allows more extensive examination of the small intestine through sequential inflation and deflation of two balloons near the tip of the instrument. This inflation and deflation helps to propel the tip of the instrument along the small intestine. The technique can be performed through the mouth, esophagus, and stomach into the first part of the small intestine, or it can be performed through the colon into the last part of the small intestine. It tends to be a longer procedure than standard endoscopy and typically requires general anesthetic or propofol for deep sedation. Using this technique, it is often possible to examine the entire length of small intestine that cannot be examined by gastroscopy or colonoscopy. Biopsies can be obtained of the inner lining of the small intestine, and the rate of progress through the small intestine is under the control of the physician, as opposed to the wireless capsule endoscopy, where the progress through the intestinal tract is largely determined by contractions of the small intestine.

Biopsies

Endoscopy also allows the operator to perform biopsies of the inner lining of the gastrointestinal tract. Small samples are taken with a tiny instrument with small jaws that can cut or pull off pieces of the inner lining. This part of the procedure is not painful; usually, the patient is not aware that it is happening. The biopsy process is very safe; complications, such as serious bleeding, are extremely uncommon.

Rule Out Other Conditions

Biopsies are usually taken to confirm the suspected diagnosis of IBD and to help rule out other conditions, such as infection. As surprising as it may seem, biopsies do not always provide 100% certainty about the diagnosis, particularly when distinguishing between Crohn's disease and ulcerative colitis. Other information, such as the location of the inflammation or other associated features, provides more assistance in diagnosis.

In some instances, biopsies are done to screen for pre-cancerous changes. Some patients with IBD involving the large intestine for more than 8 to 10 years are at increased risk of colon cancer, and their physicians may recommend a surveillance program that involves regular colonoscopy with many biopsies taken throughout the colon.

Prognosis

Once the diagnosis of IBD has been confirmed using one or more of the available investigations, some of that information can be used to help the physician determine the severity and prognosis of a patient's particular IBD. However, even with the most complete diagnostic staging, the ultimate prognosis can be unpredictable, varying from person to person with the same disorder. Patients naturally have many pressing questions about the course of their disease, which are asked and answered in the next chapter.

CHAPTER 3

What Can I Expect Now That I Have IBD?

CASE STUDY Kelly

After asking her doctor a host of questions about the symptoms and diagnosis of ulcerative colitis, Kelly was still upset because she knows of a boy who went to her high school who had ulcerative colitis. Her recollection of him was that he was sick for many days at a time. He finally had to take several weeks off school and have surgery. She is concerned that a similar fate awaits her and that she will fall behind in her university studies — or possibly even have to drop out. Even worse, she fears she may have to wear a bag to collect her stool. She has heard that people with colitis live shorter lives and are likely to develop colon cancer.

From her doctor, Kelly wants to know if the disease will get worse. What are the chances of her getting better? Will she require surgery and need a bag to collect her stool? Will she be able to live a full, productive life — complete her studies, go to work, have a family? Can she expect to live a normal life? Can she travel? And most urgently, can she die from IBD?

Again, her doctor set out to give her the information she needed to cope with her uncertainties and anxieties. Every person with IBD is unique, he told her. Just because someone she knows had a difficult time does not mean that she necessarily will. IBD is not a fatal condition, he assured her, and the majority of individuals with IBD lead productive lives — they are able to complete their studies, go to work, and have a family.

Kelly had many more questions to ask, but for now, her doctor provided her with some links to some valuable and credible websites, while cautioning her against relying on websites from unrecognized sources and discussing her disease with others in Internet chat rooms or bulletin boards. If she ever felt concerned about the reliability of the information she was finding from any source, he welcomed her to discuss it with him.

(continued on page 211)

Frequently Asked Questions

If you or a member of your family has been recently diagnosed with inflammatory bowel disease, you will likely have a number of puzzling questions, concerns, thoughts, and feelings about this condition. Different individuals have different ways of responding to bad news. For some people, there will be fear and anxiety; for others, there will be anger; for still others, there will be sadness. Some will take the news in stride, seeing the disease as a challenge, an obstacle that needs to be overcome like any other challenge they might encounter day to day. Some people will try to deny their illness or try to minimize its significance. None of these feelings or approaches to coping with disease is wrong, as long as it does not prevent the IBD sufferer from obtaining advice and care from medical professionals.

In most cases, you will know very little about the disease, which is to be expected, since most of us, unless we work in the health-care field or have a friend or relative with IBD, may not have even heard about these disorders. You will probably want to ask a number of very specific questions, even if you already know someone with IBD or if you have learned about IBD through some other means. Ask your doctor all the questions that come to mind. The answers to common questions about the course and prognosis of IBD are addressed in this chapter.

Coping with Knowledge

One way of coping with this disease is to learn as much as possible about it. In most instances, this will help you to reduce fear and anxiety, even anger and sadness.

Frequently Asked Questions about Prognosis

- Can I die from this disease?
- Will the disease get worse?
- Can my condition improve?
- Can I still go to school?
- Can I get and keep a job?
- Will I need to be hospitalized?
- Will I need to have surgery?
- Will I need a "bag" outside my body to collect stool?
- What lifestyle changes will I need to make?
- Will I be able to become pregnant?
- Can I take my medication during pregnancy?
- Will my condition flare during pregnancy?
- Will this disease affect the birth of my child?
- Can I travel if I have IBD?

Can I Die from This Disease?

Life Expectancy

Fortunately, death due to IBD is a rare occurrence and, on average, the life expectancy of people with IBD appears to be pretty much the same as people without IBD.

When someone is diagnosed with inflammatory bowel disease, the first thought that may enter the mind is "Can I die from this disease?" With improvements in the medical and surgical management of IBD, death as a result of IBD or one of its complications is exceedingly rare today, nor is life expectancy shortened.

While some older studies from the 1950s, 1960s, and 1970s suggest that the risk of dying is increased in people with IBD, these studies examined patients who had the disease before many of the modern advances in the medical and surgical care of IBD patients existed, which may have accounted for the slightly higher mortality rate. However, there does appear to be an increased mortality risk in the first year after diagnosis.

In some instances, surgery may be delayed unnecessarily, leading to more complications and, ultimately, death. Doctors, patients, and their families are sometimes reluctant to consider surgery at the time of diagnosis, even when it may be the most appropriate way of managing the disease if it is very severe. This reluctance may be partly due to the feeling on the part of the doctor that medication should be given a chance to work. Because the patient and the family are not yet familiar with the disease, they may not have come to terms with the need for surgery.

First-Year Risk

Recent studies have suggested that there may still be a slight increased risk of dying in the first year after diagnosis, but after the first year, the risk appears to be no different than in someone without IBD. The reason for this increased risk of dying in the first year after diagnosis is not very clear, but it may be due to the fact that some individuals with IBD will first present with very sudden onset of severe symptoms and severe inflammation, with the result that the correct diagnosis may not be made soon enough to begin proper treatment.

Will the Disease Get Worse?

Predicting the course of the disease in a given individual is very difficult. However, this is something that almost every patient who has been recently diagnosed with IBD wants to know.

Both Crohn's disease and ulcerative colitis are chronic, lifelong disorders that have a tendency to fluctuate in severity over time. The disease seemingly gets better or worse on its own for no apparent reason. It is not uncommon for a person with IBD to be quite well for a period of months or years, only to experience a flare or recurrence of symptoms over a period of days to weeks. Similarly, some people go on for many months or, in some cases, for years with chronic symptoms that do not respond to treatment, only to find that for some reason the symptoms begin to improve on their own.

Risk Profiles

The use of steroid medication for the first flare of disease tends to predict a poorer prognosis. However, this higher risk is probably not entirely due to the medication itself worsening the prognosis; rather, the fact that the doctor chose to use this potent medication indicates that the disease is, in the doctor's overall opinion, relatively severe and requires this medication to treat. In forming this opinion, your doctor typically uses a number of clinical clues based on their experience that tells them that the patient's disease is more severe and more likely to develop complications or require surgery.

How these clues can help predict the prognosis, for an individual patient, with a high degree of reliability has been the subject of much research. It seems that using individual patient risk profiles, consisting of a combination of factors taken together, may provide the best chance for evaluating prognosis. These risk profiles have traditionally been based on patient factors and disease factors, such as the age of first diagnosis, location of disease, severity of the first attack, and the appearance of the intestinal lining during colonoscopy.

These work reasonably well, but probably not well enough to help patients and doctors make decisions about disease management in individual patients. More recently, attempts have been made to incorporate blood tests and genetic tests into the risk profiles of patients.

First Attack

There is no question that the severity of the first attack of IBD tends to predict the subsequent course of the disease. Not all of the subsequent flares are necessarily as severe as the first one, but they still cause symptoms, require treatment, and have a significant impact upon a person's life. Patients with first attacks that are less severe tend to have a lower risk of having subsequent flares, but the risk is still present years after the original attack.

Frequency of Flares

When a flare of the disease occurs, there is usually no particular reason that can be identified for it occurring at that particular time in the course of a person's disease. It is natural to try to attribute the flare to various events that may have occurred in someone's life or to various foods that they may have eaten. For example, if you develop a flare of Crohn's disease, you may say that it was because you were eating a lot of junk food or because you are very busy at work, under considerable stress, and not getting enough rest.

Since Crohn's disease and ulcerative colitis are quite variable in their presentation from person to person, it makes sense that the factors causing flares also vary from person to person.

Right Patient, Right Time, Right Treatment

It is likely that, over the coming years, the ability to predict disease course and prognosis in individual patients will become much more accurate, to the point that these risk profiles can be used to make management decisions in individual patients. Using this type of risk assessment will help to increase the chance that the right treatment will be used for the right patient at the right time.

First-Flare Risk

In general, patients with severe episodes of IBD, especially those whose disease is severe enough to require treatment with a steroid medication, such as prednisone, will have approximately a 50% chance of having another flare within 1 year once the steroid medication is tapered off and discontinued.

Identifying these factors requires careful observation by patient and doctor to determine what might bring on a flare. Identifying something that consistently triggers a flare in an individual can provide the opportunity to take steps to reduce that risk, steps that don't necessarily involve the use of medication. However, in many if not most instances, a specific cause or trigger for a disease flare cannot be clearly identified. Even if someone with IBD can identify something that seems to bring on a flare, there is no guarantee that avoiding that trigger or minimizing its effect will necessarily allow them to avoid the risk of a flare altogether.

Severity of Disease

Some people will have very mild disease symptoms that don't interfere with their day-to-day activities, whereas others will be almost incapacitated by the severity of the symptoms. It is difficult to predict which category someone will fall into when the disease is first diagnosed.

Similar to the risk of flares, the chance of having more aggressive or severe disease tends to be higher if the first presentation is more severe. Exceptions do occur. Someone may have a severe flare at the first presentation, but once it has settled with treatment, the disease will go into a prolonged period of remission, during which time the person may have very few or no symptoms. This scenario is more common in individuals with ulcerative colitis than with Crohn's disease.

Disease that is very limited — for example, ulcerative colitis affecting only the rectum — may not progress and worsen. In this case, the area of inflammation or disease usually remains confined to the rectum and remains stable for many years. However, in approximately 10% to 20% of patients, the inflammation will extend to involve more of the colon, and the patient may become much sicker and more symptomatic when a flare occurs.

Can My Condition Improve?

The severity of Crohn's disease and ulcerative colitis can fluctuate significantly over a period of days, weeks, and months without any apparent reason. Just as a flare can occur in someone who has been quite stable for many months or years, the symptoms of disease can mysteriously improve without any intervention on the part of the doctor and without an obvious

Increased Flare Risk

It is very difficult to attribute flares to specific life events or to specific foods. Researchers have studied this issue for many years, and no factor — not stress, not diet, not infections — consistently results in increased risk of flares or worsening of the disease.

Disease Extensiveness

The likelihood that the disease will progress or worsen depends, to some degree, on the extent of intestine involved. In general, disease that is more extensive — for example, Crohn's disease that affects long segments of both the small and large intestines — may be more likely to remain active or worsen.

Successful Treatments

Most patients experiencing a flare of ulcerative colitis or Crohn's disease require and request treatment. Patients are often given nutritional advice, with special diets being recommended in specific cases. They may also receive psychological support for managing their symptoms. Although IBD cannot be cured by drug therapy, a number of medications are helpful in reducing inflammation, reducing symptoms, and, in some cases, producing a full remission whereby the patient is free of symptoms. In some cases, surgery may be required, which often has a successful outcome in eliminating or managing symptoms. These various successful treatment strategies are discussed In detail in Part 2 of this book.

cause. Individuals with mild disease may be able to afford to take a chance and wait a little while to see if their situation improves without treatment. That being said, it is unusual for someone with severe disease to improve without any treatment.

Spontaneous Recovery

Mild flares of IBD can sometimes go away without any additional treatment. This phenomenon has been well shown in clinical studies where patients with IBD receive placebo (inactive medication) as a means of comparing a new treatment to no treatment at all. Interestingly, the studies have shown that anywhere from 5% to 30% of patients treated only with placebo will experience improvement. The improvement is not necessarily complete, leading to remission, but it does indicate that the disease can improve without medication.

There have been a number of theories proposed to explain this spontaneous improvement, but no one knows for sure what factors are behind it. Improvements that occur without medication or without the addition of new medication could be due to changes in diet or stress levels, or possibly just a natural day-to-day or week-to-week fluctuation in an individual's immune response. Researchers are working to determine why disease flares occur and how spontaneous improvements occur. This information may help to develop new ways of preventing disease flares and treating IBD.

Remission

In studies of patients with Crohn's disease and ulcerative colitis, a proportion of the patients who receive no treatment will predictably experience improvement in their symptoms, and, in some cases, this improvement may be complete (although not necessarily permanent). This spontaneous improvement is more commonly seen in individuals with mild flares or mild symptoms. Simply monitoring a patient with a very mild flare may be a reasonable management approach in some instances.

Can I Still Go to School?

No Reason to Despair

While IBD can pose challenges for students, they can be managed in cooperation with the school. There is no reason to despair or set your goals lower just because you have IBD.

Because school-age children and young adults are the ones who are often diagnosed with Crohn's disease or ulcerative colitis, these diseases can potentially interfere with getting an education.

Let your teachers know that you have IBD and explain the symptoms so they understand that you may be absent from school because of flares and doctor appointments. Teachers can accommodate students who may need to be excused during class or during an exam to go to the bathroom. If you need to be away from school for a prolonged period of time, for hospitalization or surgery, you may be able to arrange for assignments to be brought to you by friends or classmates. Some hospitals provide Internet access for patients who want to keep up on their studies. Some schools use the Internet extensively to post assignments and to provide a forum for feedback from teachers.

However, when you are sick and in hospital, you may not feel up to working or reading. Your ability to concentrate may be reduced. If you happen to be away from school for many weeks at a time and have not been able to keep up with work from home or hospital, you may require additional help from the teachers or tutors in order to catch up. In postsecondary education, because of the intensive nature of the workload and the relatively short semesters, catching up may not always be possible. In some instances, you may need to take a leave or drop some courses and make them up the following term. You can ask your doctor to write a supporting letter. Although it may take you longer to complete your degree or diploma requirements, you will be less stressed and get more rest.

Discrimination

You may fear that prospective employers will disqualify you for a job once they learn about your condition. However, you are not required to disclose illnesses or disabilities to a prospective employer, nor can the employer discriminate against someone based on a disability. In the province of Ontario, for example, the Ontario Human Rights Code prohibits discrimination in employment based on disability. In the United States, the federal disability laws forbid most employers from asking about the medical conditions of an applicant, although the United States Supreme Court has ruled that an employer can refuse to hire someone who has a chronic condition that may be made worse by the job. Precise laws and rulings vary from jurisdiction to jurisdiction, so it is best to check with human resources specialists, career or hiring coaches, or lawyers when deciding on whether to disclose your condition to a prospective employer.

A minority of students have symptoms that are severe enough or persistent enough to cause them to have to change their educational objectives. It is the unpredictability of the disease that causes IBD patients to change their school plans. Frequent disease flares in people with more severe disease can require relatively long absences from school, which can, in turn, have a negative effect on grades.

Can I Get and Keep a Job?

There are many IBD sufferers who have successfully completed their education and gone on to a variety of successful careers as teachers, executives, entrepreneurs, lawyers, professors, engineers, police officers, farmers, doctors, nurses, authors, artists, and professional athletes. IBD does not necessarily mean that you will be limited in your choice of careers or that you cannot excel at your job.

Disclosure

Employers may feel deceived if the condition is not disclosed to them during the interview process and the applicant then becomes ill or incapacitated shortly after hiring. You can take this opportunity to educate your employers about your condition, though you don't need to give the details of all of your symptoms. In the end, you have to decide for yourself how much to disclose to the employer during the job interview process.

Keep in mind the perspective of your employers. They may not know much about the condition and may wonder if it will affect your work performance, if the disease is likely to progress, if the job will impact upon your condition, and if any modification in schedule or duties is required. Be prepared to answer these questions honestly. In addition to developing a more trusting relationship with the employer, disclosure may result in a more flexible work schedule or work conditions. Alternatively, you can make it clear that you don't expect any special treatment.

Disability

Although the majority of IBD sufferers are able to get and keep good jobs, there is a small proportion who have flares so frequently, or who have some degree of symptoms almost continuously, that they are not able to work. Eventually, they may need to go on short-term or long-term disability. Sometimes they are able to resume working on a limited basis if the disease can be controlled through medical or surgical management. Some people with severe symptoms gravitate to

More Understanding

Even if disclosure is not required by law, some people with chronic medical conditions prefer to disclose their condition to the employer during the interview process. If you disclose your illness to your employers, you may find that they are more understanding when you do have to take the occasional day or two off work because of your condition.

jobs where the employer is more sympathetic to their special needs or to jobs where there may be more flexibility in work hours. Many large companies have disability counselors who help people make the transition back into the workplace on a gradual basis by finding appropriate positions and work schedules that fit with their chronic symptoms.

Fortunately, most people with IBD are able to continue working in their usual job. Surveys have shown that more than 80% are ultimately able to carry on with their usual activities. There does appear to be an increase in time missed from school or work in the first year or two after the first diagnosis of IBD, but after that, the number of days missed from work is, on average, not much different from those people who do not have IBD. However, it may take several years after diagnosis for someone to get back on track.

Success Stories

Most IBD sufferers are able to lead happy and productive lives, pursuing a career that appeals to them and fits with their abilities. These people are usually able to succeed because they see their disease as just another challenge to overcome in achieving their career goals, the same way that they need to pass a school exam, develop an innovative ad campaign, or perfect a new surgical technique. Fortunately, it is only the very rare individual who is not able to pursue their chosen career path solely because of their IBD.

Will I Need to Be Hospitalized?

In the past, hospitalization for IBD patients was very common, especially at the time of first diagnosis. In recent years, disease flares have been managed on an outpatient basis, with hospitalization reserved primarily for very severe disease flares, for complications of the disease, and for surgery. Many physicians now realize that, in most cases, hospitalization is not needed to provide effective medical therapy or to properly monitor a patient's response to therapy.

However, outpatient treatment requires more time and effort on the part of the physician and other members of the health-care team. Health-care professionals now spend more time educating patients and their families about what to expect from the therapy and what to look for in the way of side effects or potential complications. This requires close communication between the treatment team — the physician or nurse clinician — and the patient and family.

Managing Unpredictability
The unpredictability of IBD can make it very difficult for some people to deal with Crohn's disease or ulcerative colitis. Planning your day-to-day activities, let alone your life, when the possibility of a flare or worsening of the disease hangs over your head is not easy. You will need to develop ways of becoming more flexible to cope with this unpredictability.

Will I Need to Have Surgery?

On average, 20% to 34% of ulcerative colitis patients and 70% to 80% of Crohn's disease patients will require surgery at some point in the course of their disease.

The likelihood of requiring surgery depends, to a large extent, on how well the disease responds to nonsurgical treatments, such as nutritional support or medications. Surgery also depends on the severity, extent, and location of the disease. Patients and families should keep in mind that hospitalization and surgery are not the same as admitting defeat, and that many IBD sufferers go on to lead very fulfilling lives with many years free from recurrent disease following surgery.

In ulcerative colitis, surgery is said to "cure" the disease, although it does leave the individual with a different internal and, occasionally, external anatomy. There are also some risks of complications of surgery. Unfortunately, in individuals with Crohn's disease, many operations carry a risk of possible recurrence of the disease in areas of the intestine that were not affected before surgery.

> **Chances of Surgery**
>
> The need for surgery depends on the nature of the condition. For example, someone with ulcerative colitis limited to the rectum will need surgery only rarely, whereas someone with an episode of colitis involving the entire colon that is severe enough to require hospitalization will have up to a 50% chance of requiring surgery within 1 year of the flare.

Will I Need a "Bag" Outside My Body to Collect Stool?

Occasionally, the surgeon must bring part of the intestine out to the skin so that the waste material (stool) collects in a bag, a procedure known as a stoma. Two main types of stomas are performed in IBD patients: an ileostomy, which involves bringing the last part of the small intestine out to the skin; and a colostomy, which involves bringing the large intestine out to the skin. These two types of stomas are somewhat different in their appearance and function.

Many patients fear the possibility of surgery because they believe that this means that they will be left with a stoma for the rest of their lives. Fortunately, this situation is the exception rather than the rule. The stoma can be reversed by another operation several months after the first. Even when a permanent stoma is required, a person can lead a normal life with good health and an active lifestyle. This requires some adjustment and support, but it can almost always be achieved.

> **Stoma**
>
> The majority of IBD surgery does not require a stoma, and when a stoma is needed, it is often temporary.

What Lifestyle Changes Will I Need to Make?

Main Lifestyle Factors

Certain lifestyle factors will increase the likelihood that a flare of IBD will occur. The main factors that can potentially lead to a flare are stress and use of non-steroidal anti-inflammatory drugs. There is more to a disease flare or worsening than a single factor. It is likely that several factors, many of which we probably don't fully understand, work together to increase the likelihood of a flare.

Stress, fatigue, colds, flu, medications, smoking, alcohol, and other lifestyle factors appear to have an impact upon Crohn's disease and ulcerative colitis. Although researchers have tried to prove the connection between these factors and disease severity, it is very difficult to prove scientifically that these associations exist. How does one measure stress or fatigue? How can you be certain that the cold you had 2 weeks ago is causing your disease to flare up now? Are two or three doses of an anti-inflammatory medication taken for a headache enough to cause increased symptoms?

There is really nothing that will guarantee that a flare will occur in a given individual. You may find that you experienced a flare during final exams in your first year of university — a time of great stress for most students — but the following year, you sailed through an equally difficult exam schedule without a disease flare.

Stress and Fatigue

Stress is often associated with disturbed sleep patterns and fatigue. Fatigue can affect immune system functioning and, possibly, IBD flares. Fatigue is a symptom of IBD that can be very difficult to treat, but it is generally considered good advice to obtain sufficient sleep and rest, particularly if you feel a flare coming on.

If you are able to get a good night's sleep but still wake feeling unrested, or if you become quickly tired during the day and have to lie down, it may be that your disease is active and causing you to feel fatigue. In some cases, even minimal inflammation of the intestine — not enough to cause any other symptoms — may produce very profound fatigue. In other instances, a vitamin or mineral deficiency, such as iron, folic acid, or vitamin B12 deficiency, can lead to fatigue. In those instances, appropriate supplementation can correct the symptom.

Impaired Sleep

If you are not sleeping well, it may be because of your disease symptoms, such as frequent diarrhea at night, but if you are not sleeping well despite the absence of symptoms, you should discuss this with your doctor. Impaired sleep can be a sign of anxiety or depression, and proper treatment can improve your sleep patterns.

Smoking

Smoking has many related health risks. In addition to its deleterious effects on the lungs and heart, smoking may also be detrimental to Crohn's disease. Smoking increases the risk of Crohn's disease first developing, and once someone has Crohn's disease, it may make the disease more aggressive. Disease seems to come back more quickly and aggressively after surgery in smokers. If you are a smoker and have Crohn's disease, you can do yourself a big favor and quit. Get all of the help you can — support from family and friends (even if they are smokers and have to quit too) and from your doctor or health-care provider for referral to smoking cessation programs or prescriptions for drugs that can help you kick the habit.

However, smoking actually appears to be protective against developing ulcerative colitis. For patients with ulcerative colitis who are former smokers, the period soon after smoking cessation seems to be a time of particularly increased risk of developing this disease. In the occasional ulcerative colitis patient who happens to be a smoker, the disease may become more active after smoking cessation. This observation has even led some researchers to use nicotine, in the form of skin patches, as a treatment for ulcerative colitis.

Despite the strong association between cigarette smoking and protection against ulcerative colitis, this approach to treatment has not been proven to be consistently effective. If you are a nonsmoker and you develop ulcerative colitis, don't start smoking, because other health risks outweigh any possible benefit that you might get from smoking.

Will I Be Able to Become Pregnant?

If your condition is under good control, you should expect to have as much chance of getting pregnant as a woman who does not have IBD. However, when the disease is active, it can get in the way of pregnancy.

If you are quite sick with a disease flare, you probably don't feel like becoming pregnant — and you may not be able to. Your symptoms and any resulting weight loss can interrupt your normal menstrual cycle, so that your ovaries may not be releasing an egg every month. If there are no eggs being released, there can be no pregnancy. Fortunately, when you recover from a flare of IBD, the menstrual cycle tends to become more regular again, the ovulation (release of eggs) resumes, and pregnancy is possible.

Surgery for IBD or complications of IBD, particularly abscesses from Crohn's disease, can lead to increased rates of infertility, probably due to scarring around the fallopian tubes, which carry the egg from the ovary to the uterus. Complications of surgery, such as a leak or an abscess, increase the rate of fertility problems even further.

> **Caution Before Surgery**
>
> Before any surgery for IBD or its complications, be sure to inform your surgeon about your plans for having children and ask what procedure would best meet your needs.

Although disease flares tend to make becoming pregnant more difficult, it is not a guarantee that you will not become pregnant. If you are sexually active during a disease flare and do not want to be pregnant, you should use appropriate birth control methods.

Can I Take My Medication during Pregnancy?

Avoid Methotrexate

If you are considering becoming pregnant, you should not take methotrexate, and if you are pregnant, you should not start methotrexate. Methotrexate has been proven to cause spontaneous abortions and malformations of the fetus.

Most medications that are used for the treatment of IBD can be used during pregnancy if they are truly needed to bring the disease under control or to maintain remission in someone who has had a very rocky course. However, do not take methotrexate. There is also some concern about the use of ciprofloxacin and its effect on cartilage development in the fetus. By all means, the 5-ASA-containing medications and steroids, such as prednisone, can be used during pregnancy and appear to be exceedingly safe with respect to their effects on the fetus and the mother.

A number of new and effective medications have become available for the treatment of IBD over the past few years, and there are likely to be more in the coming years. Although this is great news for IBD sufferers, the fact that these treatments are so new makes it impossible to know for certain what the risk of taking them during pregnancy might be, and whether they should be avoided or stopped during pregnancy. However, as time passes, more and more pregnant women will try these new treatments and we will become more familiar with what their benefits during pregnancy might be and, on the flip side, what their risks to the unborn baby might be.

Questions about medications should ideally by brought up with your doctor well before you become pregnant so that you can have a full discussion of the options available and make an informed decision about your course of action during pregnancy.

During your pregnancy, you should be followed closely by a gastroenterologist or other expert in IBD, as well as an obstetrician. Some health centers have high-risk obstetrics units for pregnant women with chronic underlying medical conditions, such as Crohn's disease or ulcerative colitis.

Will My Condition Flare during Pregnancy?

If the disease is active when you become pregnant, there is a high likelihood that it will remain active throughout the pregnancy. However, there is a significant proportion of women who say that they "never felt as well" as they did when they were pregnant. Many of them say that they wish they could figure out how to be pregnant all of the time so that their IBD remains under control. If the disease is in remission at the beginning of the pregnancy, but becomes active later on during pregnancy, it can be treated as needed with most medications normally used in nonpregnant women, with the exception of methotrexate. As discussed earlier, there may be limited information about the safety and effectiveness of newer medications in pregnancy, so they should be used only after a full discussion with your doctor that includes the potential alternatives.

> **Pregnancy Precaution**
>
> It is always best to become pregnant when your IBD is well controlled. If you do, there is a very good chance that it will remain well controlled throughout the pregnancy.

Will This Disease Affect the Birth of My Child?

Women with IBD are usually able to carry the baby to term, although there does seem to be a slightly higher rate of early or premature delivery in IBD patients, particularly if the disease is active during pregnancy. In addition, there is also a tendency to have babies that are slightly small for their gestational age.

Episiotomies are perfectly fine if they avoid an uncontrolled tear into the anal sphincter or rectum. The only time when a caesarean section might be considered solely because of the IBD and not for obstetrical reasons is in a woman with Crohn's disease who has complicated perianal disease with a lot of inflammation and possible infection around the anus and the vagina. In that particular situation, a caesarean section is probably the safest way to go.

If you have IBD, you can expect to have as much chance as any other woman of having a vaginal delivery. However, it is important for the delivering obstetrician to be aware that you have IBD and to avoid an uncontrolled tear.

Can I Travel If I Have IBD?

Traveling for business or pleasure and visiting with friends and family members far from home can often be stressful for IBD sufferers. When you are feeling well and your IBD is well controlled, you shouldn't feel hindered in your travel. If the disease is active or has been quite unpredictable, you might be best to delay your travel plans if at all possible until things are more stable. There is nothing worse than having to spend most of your time on vacation inside a hotel room because you are experiencing symptoms of IBD.

Travel R$_x$

Certain precautions and preparations need to be undertaken when you are traveling with IBD. These will vary from individual to individual, depending on the severity of the disease, its symptoms and complications, the medications being taken, and the presence of a stoma bag.

- If you are not traveling alone, try to choose traveling companions who understand your disease and the symptoms you might experience. Be honest with them. For example, you can tell them, "I have to make sure that I have a bathroom break at least every 2 hours." The travel itinerary can be planned accordingly.

- If you are traveling by plane, try to plan your bathroom visits away from times when the bathroom is busiest — usually after meals or first thing in the morning on overnight flights. Try to use the bathroom just before getting on a plane, train, or bus or before getting into a lineup at the check-in counter, security, or customs. Some people find it helpful to take an antidiarrheal medication, such as Imodium or Lomotil, just before boarding or before going on a long car trip. This can reduce the amount of diarrhea and urgency, providing some feeling of security. However, this is not safe for all people with IBD or in all situations. Be sure to check with your doctor before trying this approach.

- If loss of bowel control is a possibility or something that you worry about, make sure that you have a change of clothes and have some premoistened disposable towelettes in your carry-on luggage.

- Take time to rest and to eat regular meals. Ideally, these meals should be nutritious, but this isn't always possible on the road. When on an airplane, it is sometimes best to eat lightly and avoid foods and drinks containing caffeine — coffee, chocolates, and cola drinks — which can increase diarrhea.

- Make sure that you maintain an adequate fluid intake (preferably water), especially if you are feeling dehydrated and thirsty. As a general rule, approximately 6 to 8 glasses (1.5 to 2 L) a day should be adequate.

- If you are traveling by plane or across international borders and you are taking medications with you, take the medications in the original bottle or box that you obtained from the pharmacy, along with the pharmacy label indicating your name, the drug's name, and the physician's name. If you are traveling to another country, write down the generic name of the medications because the brand names are frequently different in different countries.

- If you are traveling with medication that requires needles or syringes, ask for a letter from your physician that describes your diagnosis and indicates your need for medication given by injection. This is absolutely necessary if you are planning on taking the medication and supplies with you as a carry-on onto an airplane. This also pertains to supplies for an ostomy.

- Ensure that your medications are not exposed to extreme temperatures (hot or cold) for prolonged periods. The same goes for stoma supplies. If you are traveling by car, don't leave the medication or supplies in the trunk or in the back seat of the car on a hot summer day or a frigid winter day. If you have medication that requires cold storage, consider the use of an insulated carrying bag with freezer packs.

- Take more medication and supplies with you than you think you will need. Some people like to pack some in their checked luggage and keep some in their carry-on luggage.

Not only do IBD symptoms make you feel bad, but you will probably feel doubly bad because you are missing out on fun and good times. That is not to say you should not travel out of fear that a flare might occur while you are away; instead, you should try to choose the best time to travel based on how you are feeling and how your disease has behaved in the past. If you are not sure, you can talk to your doctor about your travel plans.

Many people with IBD find that travel, whether due to the change in routine or the change in diet, can cause changes in the way their gastrointestinal tract functions. Diarrhea, cramping, increased gas, and abdominal distension can all occur. Traveling can be quite tiring, especially if it involves long periods in a car, bus, train, or airplane or travel across many time zones. In most cases, the symptoms experienced do not necessarily represent a flare of the disease, but are something that can be experienced by anyone, whether or not they have IBD.

Traveler's Diarrhea

When you travel, you often eat food that you have not prepared yourself and you may not be sure where the food originated. As a result, there may be a chance that you can pick up "traveler's diarrhea." This is a catch-all term for a variety of different infections caused by viruses and bacteria that may be transmitted by eating contaminated food or drinking contaminated water.

There are certain countries and locations that are well known as being places where people can pick up traveler's diarrhea if they are not careful about what they eat and drink.

Traveling Precautions

Speak with your doctor about what precautions you might take against traveler's diarrhea. Some doctors will provide a prescription for a supply of antibiotics to be taken if you develop diarrhea, rectal bleeding, and fever. However, the best treatment is prevention by being careful.

Most often these are tropical destinations. Although some of the resort areas and hotels have reasonably safe food and water supplies, you should still be careful about drinking unbottled water or drinks with ice or eating salads, unpeeled fruits, and vegetables. In general, anything that is uncooked and that might have been washed with contaminated water is best to avoid. Definitely avoid eating food from street vendors.

What Causes IBD?

Although the potential impact of Crohn's disease and ulcerative colitis on your life is the most pressing concern at the time of diagnosis, you will probably also want to know how you could have possibly developed this illness. The factors that may contribute to the development of IBD and how researchers are looking for the causes of IBD are discussed in the next chapter.

> **Devastating Effects**
>
> Although traveler's diarrhea can occur in anyone, in someone with IBD, the effects can be particularly devastating. In some cases, it can lead to a flare of the IBD.

CHAPTER 4

How Did I Get This Disease?

CASE STUDY Allison

Allison is a 27-year-old woman who works as a salesperson at a retail store. She is engaged to be married. She finds this time in her life to be very exciting but also very stressful.

Her 25-year-old brother has had Crohn's disease since he was 20. Allison has generally been quite healthy, but she smokes half a pack of cigarettes a day. She has had progressive abdominal cramps, rectal bleeding, and diarrhea for the past 2 months. She recently went to a hospital emergency department with a painful swelling near the anus. The surgeon who examined her drained what turned out to be an abscess.

Because of her history, the surgeon referred her to a gastroenterologist, who carried out a number of tests, including a colonoscopy, and found that she had Crohn's disease of both her small and large intestines. He informed her of the diagnosis and prescribed several medications.

After the shock of the new diagnosis wore off, Allison had a number of questions, but by then she had been discharged from hospital and her next appointment with the specialist was not for another 4 weeks. She notices that two of the medications she has been prescribed are antibiotics, but she has heard from her brother that Crohn's disease is not due to an infection. However, a close friend has told her that she read that Crohn's disease is caused by an unusual type of tuberculosis and can be cured by taking antibiotics against tuberculosis.

Allison wonders what has actually caused her to develop Crohn's disease. Is it an infection? Could stress have played a role? Because her brother also has Crohn's disease, could it be genetic? Could it be something in the food that they ate when they were children? Could it be due to the food she eats now? Could it be related somehow to the fact that she smokes cigarettes? The list of possible causes seemed endless.

Research Models

There are many methods by which researchers work to uncover the causes of IBD and discover why it occurs in certain individuals and not in others:

- Experiments done in test tubes using single cells or cells grown in a culture
- Experiments done in animals that develop IBD either spontaneously or through some type of experimental manipulation
- Experiments done on genetic samples taken from humans
- Experiments done on bacteria present in the intestines of IBD patients
- Experiments testing different treatment approaches in humans
- Research studies looking at factors that may predict who does and who doesn't get IBD
- Studies examining environmental factors, such as geographic location, diet, intestinal bacteria, and chemical exposures, to name a few, that might promote or protect against the development of IBD

Several theories about the cause of IBD and the intestinal inflammation process have emerged since Crohn's disease and ulcerative colitis were first described:

- IBD is an infection
- IBD is an inherited or acquired immune deficiency
- IBD is an overactive immune system acting against itself (autoimmunity)
- IBD is a reaction to some recognized or unrecognized factor in the environment
- IBD is a genetic disorder

Although researchers often believe that their own method of research will uncover the causes of IBD and, ultimately, the cure, the various methods really complement one another. It is highly likely that IBD will be found to be due to multiple factors — both those that we inherit from our parents (genetic factors) and those that we are exposed to in the food we eat, the infections we acquire, and the chemicals and toxins we may be exposed to (environmental factors).

Causal Factors

When patients are told that they have inflammatory bowel disease, the first question they will likely ask is "What is this disease?" The next question that is foremost in most people's minds concerns their pressing symptoms and their prognosis. Once the diagnosis of IBD is confirmed and the prognosis understood, they begin to question "How did I get this disease?"

Logically, understanding the causes of the disease should lead to developing a "cure." However, the causes of inflammatory bowel disease have not been determined conclusively. There appear to be a number of causal factors — and a number of corresponding treatments.

Although there have been major advances in our understanding of what happens when the bowel becomes inflamed in inflammatory bowel disease, we still do not know exactly what causes this condition. We also do not know what triggers the process of intestinal inflammation or why one person may develop it whereas a neighbor, brother, sister, or child may not. This apparent lack of research progress can be frustrating for patients and their families.

However, there has been no lack of effort to crack the mysteries of Crohn's disease and ulcerative colitis. From these research studies, we have come to recognize that there may not be a single cause that explains every manifestation of inflammatory bowel disease in every individual; instead, the disease may have many causes that interact to produce IBD in a previously healthy individual.

Possible Infectious Causes

There are many similarities between the way IBD presents in the intestines and a number of specific infections caused by bacteria, viruses, and parasites. Well-recognized intestinal infections, caused by specific bacteria (such as salmonella, campylobacter, yersinia, several strains of E. coli), by specific viruses (such as Norwalk virus and rotavirus), and by parasites (such as *Entamoeba histolytica* and giardia), often produce intestinal inflammation and damage, along with the associated symptoms of abdominal pain, diarrhea, and rectal bleeding, but they do not usually last more than several days before they are cleared by the body's immune system. These microbes (bacteria, viruses, and parasites) typically do not produce chronic or long-lasting intestinal inflammation and have not been found in the intestines or stools of patients with IBD. They usually do not recur once the microbe is cleared by the immune system, unless a person is exposed again to the microbe in question.

Bacteria

Although it appears unlikely that a disease-causing (pathogenic) bacterium is the cause of IBD, the thousands of billions of bacteria from the hundreds of bacteria species normally present in the intestine may somehow contribute to the inflammatory process. No single bacterial species or strain is solely responsible for the inflammatory effect; it requires a particular combination of strains to induce inflammation in someone who is genetically susceptible.

Clostridium difficile

One particular bacterial infection, called *Clostridium difficile*, is found in the stool of IBD patients from time to time, particularly during a flare of the disease. However, *Clostridium difficile* is not known to cause IBD; rather, IBD likely provides suitable conditions for the growth of this bacterial species.

L-Forms

Other bacteria that do not cause infection may contribute to the cause of IBD. Researchers have experimented with bacteria that were missing their cell wall as a possible cause. It was thought that these bacteria, called L-forms, could produce chronic infection that is indistinguishable from IBD. Subsequent studies have shown that these bacterial forms are not involved in IBD.

Mycobacteria

Another species of mycobacterium, called *Mycobacterium paratuberculosis*, produces Johne's disease in cattle. Johne's disease looks somewhat like Crohn's disease in humans. Prevalent in dairy herds and excreted in milk from infected cows, this bacterium is not completely killed by the pasteurization of milk and is, therefore, potentially present in the milk supply. Some experts have suggested that *Mycobacterium paratuberculosis* may be able to infect humans and that this chronic infection may be the cause of Crohn's disease, in at least some patients.

In some studies, researchers have been able to detect antibodies against specific segments of mycobacterial proteins in the blood of human Crohn's disease patients, and in other studies, they have been able to detect genetic sequences specific to mycobacteria in inflamed intestinal tissues of Crohn's disease patients.

Some investigators have apparently had success in treating Crohn's disease using regimens consisting of multiple antibiotics that are active against *Mycobacterium paratuberculosis*. However, the number of patients treated has been relatively small, and most researchers have not been able to reproduce the findings of mycobacteria in the intestinal tissues or the response to therapy against mycobacteria.

> **Tuberculosis**
>
> Some researchers have suggested that the bacteria causing tuberculosis in humans might be the cause of Crohn's disease. *Mycobacterium tuberculosis* can infect the intestines, and the appearance of Crohn's disease has some similarities to intestinal tuberculosis. However, careful study of intestinal tissues from Crohn's disease patients has not shown tuberculosis infection to be a cause.

Viruses

Microbes other than bacteria can cause intestinal inflammation and have, therefore, also been considered as possible causes of IBD. Viruses, in particular, may be very difficult to detect in the intestinal lining or in stool samples, and it has been speculated that a virus that has eluded detection may be the cause of IBD.

Paramyxoviruses (Measles)

Paramyxoviruses, of which the measles virus is the best known, has received considerable attention. By using blood testing to detect antibodies directed against paramyxovirus or by using very powerful electron microscopy on biopsy and surgical resection specimens, some investigators have found what they believe to be evidence of a paramyxovirus infection in Crohn's disease patients. However, more recent studies using very sensitive genetic probes for paramyxovirus have not been able to detect this evidence of measles virus.

Subsequently, the proponents of the "measles theory" have suggested that it is not necessarily an actual infection by measles virus that produces Crohn's disease, but rather the late effects of early childhood infection or exposure of one's mother to measles virus during pregnancy. They have also suggested that Crohn's disease may be a result of childhood immunization against measles using the live measles vaccine, in which the virus is still alive but cannot produce the usual measles infection. There is some indirect evidence supporting this theory, but it consists mainly of the apparent increase in the incidence of Crohn's disease following the institution of universal measles vaccination programs in developed countries in the 1960s. The weight of the evidence supports the conclusion that IBD is not due to measles infection, exposure, or vaccination.

Possible Environmental Causes

There are differences in the prevalence of Crohn's disease and ulcerative colitis between countries, as well as between ethnic groups within a given country. These differences have led scientists to suggest that, in addition to infections, other environmental factors, such as toxins, diet, smoking, medication use, and even geography, may have a significant influence on the development of IBD.

No Direct Viral Link

Numerous viruses have been suggested as being the possible offending agent, but none has been found consistently in the intestinal lining or stool, despite newer, more sophisticated techniques that have been used over the past 10 years.

Measles Theory

Most experts do not subscribe to the measles theory because the bulk of the evidence shows little or no suggestion of measles infection in the intestines of Crohn's disease patients and does not explain many other aspects of the changing patterns of IBD.

Twin Studies

We know that environmental factors influence IBD from studies of twins. When one identical twin has Crohn's disease or ulcerative colitis, the other twin, who is genetically identical, will not necessarily develop IBD. To produce the disease, some environmental influence or exposure must interact with the genetic background that makes a person susceptible to developing IBD. Presumably, one twin has been exposed to disease-causing environmental factors, while the other has not been exposed to those factors or has not been exposed for long enough or exposed at the right time in the course of growth and development.

Population Studies

Researchers have tried to determine what some of these environmental factors might be in a number of ways. Often, they will take a group of IBD patients and find out about various possible risk factors that they might have been exposed to and compare them to a group of similar individuals who do not have IBD. Researchers will also examine where people with IBD were born and where they grew up, while looking for clues to possible environmental exposures.

Through these studies, it has been discovered that the incidence of IBD is highest in developed North American and Northern European countries and lower in less developed or more southerly countries. This has raised the theory that something we are exposed to in developed countries contributes to the development of IBD. An interesting observation is the change in the pattern of IBD in other areas of the world. In Japan, for example, Crohn's disease was almost unheard of in 1950, but the incidence of the disease has risen steadily since then. This increase has been explained by some experts as the result of a change in the Japanese diet. During the time that Crohn's disease has increased in Japan, the diet has become increasingly Westernized, with less traditional rice and fish and more red meat being eaten. However, the change in diet and the increase in incidence do not prove cause and effect, since many other aspects of life in Japan changed between 1950 and the present time.

Diet

Dietary factors are obvious potential risk factors, given that Crohn's disease and ulcerative colitis are intestinal disorders. Food comes into direct contact with the intestinal

Environmental Triggers

IBD patients may experience spontaneous improvements and relapses. However, we do not know what induces or triggers a change in the degree of inflammation in the intestines. Despite extensive research, we cannot say for certain what environmental factors may trigger the disease initially or may result in exacerbations once the disease is established.

Breastfeeding Protection

Children who have been breastfed may be at lower risk of subsequently developing IBD than children who have been formula-fed. If true, this would mean that there is something potentially harmful in infant formula or, more likely, something protective in breast milk.

lining. Although no specific food or food category has been consistently found to be a potential triggering factor in IBD, some studies have found that diets that are high in red meat or refined sugars may increase the risk of developing IBD.

Altering dietary intake may result in improvement in intestinal inflammation and symptoms of disease. This is not to say that dietary factors cause IBD, but once IBD is established, modification of the diet may, in some instances, improve the disease activity and symptoms.

There may be some factor in the diet that worsens or propagates the inflammatory reaction in the intestines of IBD patients. It is not clear what this factor or factors might be. Attempts at carrying out exclusion or elimination diets, in which specific foods are removed from and then added back into the diet one at a time, have not identified a specific food trigger in the majority of patients.

Hygiene

In recent years, there has been interest in the so-called hygiene hypothesis to explain a number of chronic inflammatory or autoimmune diseases, such as asthma. As a result of living in an increasingly clean and hygienic society, we are not exposed to many of the infections that we once were. This is particularly true in the early childhood years. As a result, a person's immune system may become overactive because it is not accustomed to dealing with bacteria, viruses, and parasites. This leads to increased immune or inflammatory responses to proteins, bacteria, and viruses that would not have been considered "foreign" or would not have produced such a vigorous and damaging response in the past.

Environmental Exposures

Since the appearance of IBD seems to have coincided with the advent of modern industrialized society, other aspects of our modern society are being explored as important environmental factors that have, in some way, contributed to the rise in IBD. Prominent among these are airborne environmental pollutants caused by internal combustion vehicles and by industry. Studies investigating the numerous possible environmental exposures are still at a relatively early stage, but there are certain environmental pollutants or toxins that theoretically may have an impact upon the immune system.

Smoking

The relationship between cigarette smoking and IBD has long been known. Patients with ulcerative colitis are more likely to be nonsmokers or former smokers, and patients with Crohn's disease are more likely to be smokers. How cigarette smoking interacts with other factors to either increase or decrease the risk of disease is entirely unknown.

Medications

Some medications are known to cause irritation and even damage to the lining of the intestinal tract. Aspirin and nonsteroidal anti-inflammatory drugs (for example, ibuprofen, naproxen, diclofenac, and sulindac) are well known to cause ulcers in the stomach and duodenum. These drugs can also have damaging effects on the lining of the intestinal tract in the last part of the small intestine (ileum) and the large intestine, the areas most commonly affected in IBD.

Antibiotics have been attracting considerable attention as a possible contributor to the onset of IBD. In particular, the use of antibiotics in early childhood has been associated in some studies with an increased risk of developing IBD in later childhood or even in adolescence or early adult life. One theory as to why that might be is that use of antibiotics in early life may have an impact on the type and variety of bacteria that are normally present in our intestines, and this change in our bacteria may affect our risk of developing IBD.

> **No Drug Cause**
>
> Despite the potential for tissue damage and the risk of a flare when using aspirin and nonsteroidal anti-inflammatory drugs, these drugs have not been shown to cause Crohn's disease or ulcerative colitis.

Possible Inherited (Genetic) Factors

Crohn's disease and ulcerative colitis have a tendency to run in families. This inherited susceptibility to the disease is carried within the genetic code. The genetic code is present, at some point in development, in every cell of the human body and is passed down from parent to child. Recent research has shown that there are over 200 inherited susceptibility factors (genes) that, when altered, can increase a person's chances of developing inflammatory bowel disease. Some of these genes appear to be specific to Crohn's disease risk, some appear to be specific to ulcerative colitis, and some appear to be shared by the two disorders.

Gene Basics

Genes contain the code that determines most of the physical characteristics of a person, animal, or plant. Not only do genes determine a person's height, hair and eye color, and blood type, they also determine a person's susceptibility to developing a wide range of diseases and disorders.

- Genes are made up of a molecule called deoxyribonucleic acid (DNA). There are tens of thousands of genes in every human being, each one coded for one of tens of thousands of corresponding proteins that are produced by the cells and tissues of a person. Through these protein products, the genes are able to determine a person's physical characteristics or disease susceptibility.

- Each gene is made up of a series of molecule fragments, called bases. The sequence of these bases — there are four bases in total, represented by the letters A, T, C, and G — tells the body how to make the protein in question. If one or more of these letters are missing or out of order, or if one or more extra letters are present in the wrong place (also known as mutations), the protein that is produced may be defective or it may not be produced at all.

- Each person has two copies of each gene — one inherited from the mother and one inherited from the father. Some diseases require just one of the two copies to be abnormal in order to produce disease, whereas other diseases require both copies to be abnormal. In some diseases, the risk is increased only slightly with one abnormal copy and increased to a much greater extent when two abnormal copies are present.

Genetic Risk

Approximately 10% to 20% of individuals with IBD have another affected family member. If someone within a family has Crohn's disease or ulcerative colitis, the chance of an unaffected member of the family developing IBD is as high as 10%, depending on the nature of the relationship and whether the individual has Crohn's disease or ulcerative colitis. In general, Crohn's disease appears to have a greater tendency to run in families.

Human Genome

Researchers have identified over 200 gene variations that appear to influence the likelihood of developing Crohn's disease or ulcerative colitis. Some seem to be specific to Crohn's disease, some appear to be more specific to ulcerative colitis, and a few appear to be associated with both diseases.

- One of the major breakthroughs in the field of IBD genetics has been the discovery that a gene called NOD-2 (also referred to as CARD15) can result in susceptibility to developing Crohn's disease. When one of the two copies of the NOD-2 gene is mutated, thereby resulting in an abnormal or absent protein product, the risk of developing Crohn's disease is approximately doubled or tripled. If both copies of the NOD-2 gene are abnormal, the risk of developing Crohn's disease is as much as 30 times greater than if both copies of the gene are normal.

- There are three common abnormalities of the NOD-2 gene, any one of which can result in the increased risk. Mutations in the NOD-2 gene may be responsible for as much as 20% of Crohn's disease in populations of European background. When the NOD-2 gene is abnormal, various cells in the body, in particular immune reactive cells, can produce either an abnormal version of the NOD-2 protein or they don't produce the NOD-2 protein at all.

- The NOD-2 gene product appears to be involved in the part of a person's immune response that is important in fighting off certain bacterial infections or responding to the by-products of certain bacteria. This may mean that NOD-2 gene mutations can cause a disruption of this part of the immune response to bacteria. This may lead to an abnormal interaction between the human host and the bacteria in the intestines. This abnormal interaction may then lead to uncontrolled intestinal inflammation and IBD.

- Some of the other genes that have been possibly linked to the development of IBD may be involved in maintaining the barrier function of the intestinal lining. When the barrier function of the intestine is defective, it may be possible for large molecules, such as proteins and intestinal bacteria, to cross into the bowel wall. These proteins and bacteria, which are considered to be "foreign" by the person's immune system, can then cause an inflammatory reaction. This inflammatory reaction is normally intended to eliminate the foreign protein or bacteria, but in IBD, the reaction is not properly controlled or regulated.

- Other genes associated with IBD are, like the NOD-2/CARD15 gene, responsible for the response to bacteria. Another group of genes is responsible for the process of cellular "housekeeping," which results in elimination of debris within cells and also causes old or damaged cells to undergo elimination. Yet another group of genes associated with IBD is responsible for various aspects of the body's immune response.

Q What is the risk to a brother or sister of a person with IBD?

A When a person has Crohn's disease, siblings have an approximately 1 in 12 chance of developing inflammatory bowel disease, either Crohn's disease or ulcerative colitis, in their lifetime. The risk of developing Crohn's disease is probably 5 times that of ulcerative colitis. When a person has ulcerative colitis, siblings have approximately a 1 in 20 chance of developing IBD in their lifetime. In that instance, the risk of ulcerative colitis is likely twice the risk of Crohn's disease.

Q What is the risk to a child of a mother or father with IBD?

A When a father or mother has Crohn's disease, their children have approximately a 1 in 15 chance of developing IBD in their lifetime. The risk is 3 to 5 times higher when the parent has Crohn's disease rather than ulcerative colitis. When a parent has ulcerative colitis, the children have approximately a 1 in 25 chance of developing IBD in their lifetime. When the parent has ulcerative colitis, the type of IBD that a child may develop is more likely to be ulcerative colitis than it is to be Crohn's disease. In that instance, ulcerative colitis is approximately twice as likely as Crohn's disease.

It does not seem to matter whether it is the father or mother who has IBD when discussing the risk to the child. The disease can be passed down from either parent. When both parents have IBD, which is unusual, the children have a much higher risk of developing IBD than would be the case if only one parent has IBD. While it is difficult to provide an exact estimate of what this risk to a child of two affected parents would be, it is probably more than 1 chance in 10 and possibly as much as 1 chance in 3.

Q **What is the risk to a parent of a person with IBD?**

A Although the risk to a parent is very low if a child has IBD, it is still higher than it would be if the mother or father didn't have any family history of IBD. In most instances where a child and parent both have IBD, the parent has usually developed the disease first, and the child has developed the disease some time after it has developed in the parent. This is usually many years later.

Q **I have IBD... what can I do to prevent my child from developing IBD in the future?**

A Although a family history of IBD involving a parent or a sibling is the strongest known risk factor for developing the disease, there really is not much that can be done to prevent the development of the disease in a child or a sibling of a person with IBD.

This is primarily because we do not know exactly what triggers the development of IBD in a person who is at risk. We also do not know how the possible risk factors that individuals might be exposed to will interact with their genetic makeup. Some environmental factors may be protective in individuals with a certain genetic makeup and may increase risk of disease in other individuals with another genetic makeup. An example of this is the effect of cigarette smoking, which seems to protect against the development of ulcerative colitis, whereas it may increase the risk of Crohn's disease or, possibly, make the course of disease more severe.

No Guarantees

Children of a parent with IBD are much more likely not to develop IBD in their lifetime than they are to develop the disease. In other words, the presence of a positive genetic test or genetic risk factor, such as a family history of IBD, does not equal the presence of IBD. Likewise, a negative result on the current genetic risk markers does not guarantee that IBD will not develop in the future.

Twin Studies

In studies of twins, in which at least one twin has IBD, it has been found that if one twin has Crohn's disease, the likelihood that the other twin also has Crohn's disease is much higher if the twins are genetically identical than if the twins are not genetically identical (fraternal twins). Since both identical twins and fraternal twins tend to share the same non-inherited factors, such as diet and environmental exposures, the higher risk in identical twins means that a genetic, or inherited, factor must be playing an important role in causing disease susceptibility.

Multiple Genes

By examining the patterns of IBD inheritance in families, it is clear that Crohn's disease and ulcerative colitis are not passed from parent to child in a simple or direct fashion the way that some physical characteristics, such as eye color, blood type, or some diseases (cystic fibrosis, for example), are passed on from parent to child. In those instances, a single gene is responsible for the particular characteristic or disease. In IBD, it appears that variations or mutations of multiple genes are required to produce increased susceptibility to the disease.

Research into the genetic factors that contribute to IBD has been exploding in the past two decades with several major successes. These successes will almost certainly lead to improved understanding of how IBD occurs and, with time, may lead to improved treatments or preventive therapy.

Is My Family at Risk?

If you or a family member has IBD, the fact that certain genes, when abnormal or altered, may lead to an increased risk of developing IBD is of some interest, particularly if such knowledge ultimately leads to more effective treatment, prevention, or even cure. However, what you really want to know is, what is the risk to other family members and is there a way to predict who might develop IBD?

The risk of developing IBD is highest in first-degree relatives (brothers, sisters, parents, and children) of an affected individual. This risk to family members is higher if the person has Crohn's disease rather than ulcerative colitis. The risks described on pages 84–85 are estimated based on the observed frequency of Crohn's disease and ulcerative colitis within families and should not be considered necessarily exact.

Genetic Counseling

Any predictive genetic testing for any disorder should ideally be accompanied by counseling from an expert physician or genetic counselor *before* the test is made. Information derived from the test may have no value for predicting disease or treating the disorder in an individual. However, this information could potentially be used by insurance companies to deny coverage or by employers to limit employment opportunities.

Genetic Testing

Unfortunately, genetic testing for IBD is not yet sensitive enough to be used as a routine tool to predict the development of disease. Even if predictive tests were more sensitive, the results may not be valuable for treating the disease for several reasons.

Possible False Symptoms

A positive genetic test in someone with a family history may make that person or family members more vigilant in watching for early signs of disease. This may unnecessarily increase anxiety around the occurrence of symptoms that are in no way related to IBD.

Possible Unnecessary Treatment

We also do not know if earlier detection of disease, even before symptoms have begun, will allow more effective treatment of acute symptoms or prevention of long-term disease complications. Early treatment of the disease, before symptoms have begun, may produce more harm than good, unless that treatment is highly effective and very safe. Current treatments for IBD are either minimally effective or are more effective but with the cost of potential side effects, some of which may be quite serious.

Despite the reservations surrounding genetic testing, it is quite likely that some people with a family history of IBD and even some without any family history will wish to have genetic testing where it is made available. Although we do not know for certain if early treatment is of benefit, many people with positive genetic tests, even without signs or symptoms of disease, will choose to receive treatment. In a survey of IBD patients, a large percentage said they would choose to have genetic testing for their children, even if a positive test had a very low likelihood of predicting disease.

Pharmacogenomics

Where genetic testing may be more widely used, at least in the next few years, is for predicting complications and the course of the disease. Genetic testing may also prove to be valuable in treating the disease, especially in choosing effective medications. This involves the science of pharmacogenomics.

Pharmacogenomics is the use of genetic testing to predict various aspects of response — both good and bad — to medications. For example, genetic testing may predict who will respond positively to a given medication and who will likely develop side effects and thus may not be a good candidate for a given medication or may require closer monitoring.

Tailored Treatments

As we become more knowledgeable about the way various drug therapies work and the genes that determine their ability to improve disease symptoms or produce side effects, we may be able to develop treatments that can be tailored specifically for individuals based on their genetic profile.

In IBD treatment, this may occur with the use of the immune modulator drugs azathioprine and 6-mercaptopurine. The way these drugs are metabolized (broken down) in the body is determined, to a large extent, by genetic factors. Most people break the drug down into inactive by-products at roughly the same rate. However, about 10% of people break the drug down slightly more slowly, and about 1% or less break the drug down very slowly. With slow drug metabolism, there may be higher levels of the active drug in the body for the same dose. Levels of the drug that are too high tend to produce toxicity to the bone marrow, resulting in the production of fewer white blood cells and the possibility of infection.

Metabolism of these drugs is determined by the level of the thiopurine methyltransferase (TPMT) enzyme in the bloodstream, which, in turn, is determined, to a large extent, by a specific genetic factor that can be detected through blood tests. By testing for the level of this enzyme in the blood, it may be possible to predict who is at risk for complications that occur as a result of high drug levels in the body. In this case, these drugs are often best avoided or, if used, given at much lower doses than would normally be used to treat IBD.

Unified Theory

Research has found no single cause or pathway to Crohn's disease or ulcerative colitis. Prevailing wisdom suggests that inflammatory bowel disease typically occurs in a genetically susceptible person when triggered by environmental factors.

Overlapping Genetic and Environmental Factors

Genetic Susceptibility — IBD — Environmental Factors (diet, infections, toxins, intestinal microbes)

No Disease

- Someone may have inherited this susceptibility without anyone else being affected in the family. Probably, a specific combination of genetic changes or mutations comes together in an individual that, in turn, leads to this increased disease susceptibility.
- In a person with this inherited susceptibility, there may be some type of environmental exposure that, if present at sufficient levels for a sufficient period of time, will trigger uncontrolled intestinal inflammation.
- The timing of this exposure, relative to the person's age, stage of development, and presence of other environmental factors, may be critical in the process leading to disease. Alternatively, there may be protective factors that, if a susceptible individual is not exposed to, will lead to a greater likelihood of developing of IBD.
- In humans, IBD can sometimes be successfully treated with antibiotic therapy. Antibiotic treatment is not necessarily killing a disease-causing bacteria; rather, it is changing the balance or composition of the normal intestinal bacterial population.

Based on these observations, you could imagine a situation in which a genetically susceptible individual develops long-lasting uncontrolled intestinal inflammation in the presence of certain normal intestinal bacteria and possibly other environmental and dietary factors. Once initiated in a genetically susceptible person, it may not be possible to shut down or decrease the uncontrolled inflammation completely. As a result, the intestine is damaged, and the symptoms of IBD become evident. In a person who is not genetically susceptible, the inflammation can be kept at levels that are sufficient to protect against infections or other outside attackers, but not so high that it would cause excessive damage to the lining of the intestine.

Intestinal Bacteria

Among environmental factors, there is considerable evidence to support the role of intestinal bacteria as being critical to the development of IBD. In almost every animal model of IBD where the role of intestinal bacteria has been studied, IBD does not develop when the experimental animals are raised in an environment that does not allow them to develop normal intestinal bacteria. If intestinal bacteria are introduced into the animal or into the environment, the animal then develops IBD.

Implications for Treatment

By following these lines of inquiry and remaining open to new discoveries, we may soon be able to identify all the pieces of this complex puzzle and, ultimately, put them together to provide a complete picture of the causes of IBD. In the meantime, there is much we can do to manage this disease successfully with diet, counseling, medications, and surgery.

PART 2

MANAGING INFLAMMATORY BOWEL DISEASE

CHAPTER 5

Dietary Strategies for Managing IBD

Julie Cepo and A. Hillary Steinhart

CASE STUDY Sabrina

Sabrina is an active 24-year-old woman who was diagnosed with Crohn's disease last year. She works during the day, but still finds time to participate in her favorite team sports and to meet with friends for dinners and movies. For the past month, Sabrina has noticed cramps and occasional abdominal pain after eating. At her friend's last barbecue, she ate steak, baked potato, and corn on the cob, but soon after, she had to leave the gathering early as a result of symptoms of abdominal bloating, cramping, and pain.

Because this had never happened before when she had eaten out, Sabrina decided to find out what she could do to improve her situation. She searched the Internet for information on any connections between diet and Crohn's disease, especially foods that might trigger flares in her disease. Friends and family offered plenty of advice about what foods she should avoid. Sabrina tried eliminating all vegetables and many fruits. She cut out red meat and dairy just in case. However, she began to lose weight quickly, enjoyed eating less, and started to stay away from get-togethers because she disliked the questions about why she was eating differently. Her cramps and pain continued despite her best efforts, so Sabrina decided it was time to make an appointment with her doctor for help.

Sabrina's health-care team provided medical therapy and answered her questions. She learned that foods don't cause or cure IBD, and that when she ate some foods, such as corn and potato skins, her symptoms worsened because these foods are difficult to digest. She was advised to follow a low-fiber diet and gradually return to her regular diet once her disease flare and symptoms resolved.

Sabrina still notices she is sensitive to some foods if they are gas-producing or she doesn't chew them well. She also understands that this type of food sensitivity is common to many people, not just those living with IBD.

Reliable Information

Nutrition is a topic of high priority not only for people living with Crohn's disease and ulcerative colitis, but also for their family and friends. Perhaps you have been diagnosed with IBD and are wondering if your current diet is appropriate. Maybe your spouse or child has been diagnosed and you are questioning if the usual foods you buy at the grocery store can still be part of your family's diet. Or maybe you've been living with IBD for a long time but are still afraid to try new foods. How can you find the answers to your questions and, at the same time, feel confident that the information you find is reliable?

Nutrition plays an important role in the management of IBD by maintaining general health during times of disease activity and during times of remission. Diet can also help with symptom management during disease flares. A person's nutritional status affects important physiological processes, such as immunity and wound healing, and, as a result, can contribute to the prevention of long-term complications. Our diet also contributes to our quality of life. Eating good-tasting food that is healthy for you should be your dietary goal, even if you have IBD symptoms. While good nutrition does not cure IBD and while, with certain exceptions, nutritional therapy does not always control disease flares, nutrition is important for health maintenance and symptom management.

Diet Studies

Diet has been studied as a possible cause of Crohn's disease and ulcerative colitis and as a possible treatment for these conditions. Although no one dietary factor has been identified as a cause of IBD, certain dietary factors could possibly play a role in increasing the risk of developing the disease or triggering a disease flare in someone who already has the disease. These factors have not been identified, and no one diet has been proven to cure IBD. Specific foods have been identified as items to avoid in managing some symptoms.

 Q **Where can I find good dietary advice?**

 A Your family doctor or gastrointestinal specialist may refer you to a registered dietitian (RD) for specific dietary advice in managing your symptoms. Registered dietitians are nutrition experts in food science who have completed a university education, as well as a nationally accredited internship program. The title "Registered Dietitian" is protected in Canada under the regulated health professionals acts, whereas the title "nutritionist" has no minimum qualifications in Canada. Similar restrictions on the use of the title "Registered Dietitian" apply in the United States.

This means that a dietitian is accountable to the public for providing reliable and safe information. Dietitians are professionals qualified to consult, assess, and evaluate nutritional status and to provide advice for preventing and treating disease. Dietitians work in health care, industry, research, and government. Look for the initials behind the professional's name: RD, RDN, P.Dt., Dt.P., and R.Dt.

Q **Did something I eat cause my IBD?**

A If doctors or dietitians knew which foods, food components, food additives, food proteins, food preservatives, or food contaminants contribute to the development of IBD, they would be the first to warn susceptible individuals to avoid them. However, to start avoiding foods without scientific evidence of the real cause of this disease is a risky practice because it can affect your relationship with food and eating, can leave you with limited choices, and can result in serious health consequences as a result of inappropriately limiting nutrients. Well-founded nutrition advice can help you to achieve better health and prevent false hope without delaying effective strategies.

The Right Diet

Statement of Liability

This chapter contains references to products that may not be available everywhere. The intent of the information provided is to be helpful; however, there is no guarantee of results associated with the information provided. Use of brand names is for educational purposes only and does not imply endorsement.

No IBD Diet

While there is no such thing as an "IBD diet," there are many foods that affect individuals living with IBD adversely or positively. There isn't any single diet that works for everyone with IBD.

Many people hear that a particular diet will help their IBD. Gaining a sense of control by changing what or how you eat can be appealing when living with an unpredictable disease. In some cases, the diet may claim to prevent disease relapse or even cure your IBD. Other diets claim to influence your immune system positively, improve digestive health, and reduce inflammation. However, just because it is in print does not mean it is true or scientifically valid.

Sometimes diets are developed in a way that has not been proven or does not even make sense physiologically. It can be difficult to sort out myth from science. A persuasive author or an impressive anecdotal story of someone whose IBD responded only to the author's diet can be very impressive and may leave you with the impression that there is some merit in what the author is suggesting. However, such anecdotes may provide false hope. The money you spend should be for reliable, evidence-based strategies. If you've had difficulty figuring out the "right" diet to follow, it is probably because your experience with diet has been different from someone else's experience.

We each have different taste preferences, different tolerances (to spicy or gas-producing foods, for example), different budgets, and even different food availability, with limited food choices in remote areas. Not only are these circumstances applicable for an individual living with IBD, there could be additional dietary considerations, including transient intolerances to previously enjoyed foods and the need to restrict some foods temporarily and supplement others. Considering these factors, it makes sense that the same food can be experienced differently by different individuals. If you then add personal tolerances and our unique likes and dislikes, there could be many thousand versions of the "right" diet.

Individualized Diets

Accordingly, all nutrition care should be individualized and developed with your doctor or registered dietitian to ensure it is realistic and successful. Remember that Crohn's disease and ulcerative colitis have different parts of the bowel that are inflamed, different disease characteristics, different disease courses, a variety of possible symptoms and possible complications, and variations in treatment regimens.

Nutrition recommendations must be balanced to avoid nutrient deficiencies and individualized to specific tastes, budgets, lifestyles, and, very importantly, for specific desired functional benefits (for example, regaining weight, symptom management). The diet that considers and meets these needs is the right diet for you.

However, there are some common dietary guidelines that people with IBD could follow in an effort to manage their symptoms and improve their quality of life — and even ward off more serious complications, such as malnutrition.

Preventing Malnutrition

Diet is the key for preventing clinical malnutrition, a condition that results when there is a deficiency or imbalance of nutrients in our body. Nutrient deficiencies can result over time from a lack of overall calories (the term "calories" can be used interchangeably with "energy") or from a lack of specific nutrients, such as protein, essential fats, vitamins, minerals, or trace elements.

Malnutrition is a concern because it can affect your immune system function, leading to an increased susceptibility to infections. It also compromises your body's normal defenses against free radicals (damaging molecules produced from pollution, radiation, stress, and smoking), slows down wound healing, and can contribute to long-term complications, such as poor dental health and early bone loss leading to osteoporosis. When you are poorly nourished, the symptoms of your IBD are likely to become more severe or have a more significant impact upon you.

Malnutrition Symptoms

Malnutrition can manifest as weight loss, loss of appetite, muscle weakness (from losing muscle mass), or changes in your skin, hair, nails, gums, eyesight, or mood.

Weight Loss

The most common indicator of malnutrition is a significant loss of body weight. Often, when you are not feeling well, you have little appetite and feel as if you must force yourself to eat. And often you still lose weight despite your efforts. Why does this happen? This is not simply a matter of willpower.

In Crohn's disease and ulcerative colitis, various parts of the gastrointestinal tract become inflamed, and although the inflammation occurs primarily at a local level (the bowel tissue), it can also occur at a whole-body, or systemic, level. Systemic inflammation results from inflammatory molecules (proteins called cytokines), which are produced in the inflamed intestine, but which circulate throughout the body. It is the effect of one or more of these cytokines that can lead to a loss of appetite.

Anorexia is one malnutrition risk factor that, along with other symptoms, such as gastrointestinal intolerance, altered taste, and dietary eliminations (food phobias and dependencies), can lead to inadequate intake. Other risk factors for malnutrition include increased nutrient requirements, malabsorption of nutrients, and increased losses of electrolytes, minerals, trace elements, and proteins. These factors can lead to malnutrition in individuals with IBD, but this doesn't mean that you will develop these symptoms or complications just because you have IBD. Also keep in mind that some are specific to either Crohn's disease or ulcerative colitis.

Treatment for Malnutrition

To determine if you are malnourished, health-care professionals will evaluate your symptoms and signs, medical history, height and weight trends, diet history, social and economic circumstances, medications, and laboratory tests. Although there are several complicated formulas that have been developed to evaluate nutritional status and nutritional risk, most physicians and dietitians can answer these questions quite easily. An appropriate nutrition plan can then be created to help manage your illness and achieve your desired health outcomes.

Your nutrition plan could include counseling for diet modifications or implementing specialized nutrition therapies. These could include help with food ideas and also supplementation with nutritional products, replacement of vitamins and minerals, provision of enteral nutrition (liquid nutrition formula delivered using a feeding tube into the stomach or small intestine), or provision of parenteral nutrition (intravenous nutrition infused through a special intravenous line).

Anorexia

Loss of appetite and the inability to eat enough to maintain your weight is described as a symptom called anorexia (this term does not mean the same as an eating disorder). Anorexia may be one of the symptoms you experience when your disease is active.

Risk Factors

If you experience symptoms or changes similar to those listed among malnutrition risk factors, be sure to mention them to your doctor. The sooner your symptoms are addressed, the less likely you are to experience the negative effects of malnutrition.

Malnutrition Risk Factors

1. Inadequate Intake of Nutrients

- **Anorexia**
  - Decreased oral intake of food and beverages
  - Inability to tolerate solid foods and a prolonged period consuming low-calorie and low-protein fluids
- **Gastrointestinal intolerance**
  - Nausea, vomiting, diarrhea, rectal urgency, cramping, bloating, pain, obstructive symptoms, pain with swallowing
- **Altered taste**
  - Side effect from some medications or a specific nutrient deficiency
- **Dietary eliminations**
  - Food phobias, food intolerances, diet experimentation
  - Dependencies (e.g., substituting alcohol for nutritious foods)

2. Increased Nutrient Requirements

- **Higher metabolic rate**
  - Stress response and inflammation, infection, wound healing, fever, catabolic (breakdown) effects from steroids
  - Increased nutrient or calorie requirements for growth (children and adolescents)
  - Repletion (building) of body tissue stores of muscle and fat

3. Malabsorption of Nutrients

- **Decreased absorptive surface**
  - Active disease affecting bowel surface
  - Multiple surgical resections
- **Nutrient bypass**
  - Fistula
  - Surgical
- **Drug interference**
- **Bile salt deficiency**
- **Small intestinal bacterial overgrowth (SIBO)**

4. Increased Losses
(electrolytes, minerals, trace elements, protein)

- **Diarrhea**
- **Fistula**
- **Blood loss**

Eating Well with Canada's Food Guide

Recommended Number of *Food Guide Servings* per Day

	Children			Teens		Adults			
Age in Years	2-3	4-8	9-13	14-18		19-50		51+	
Sex	Girls and Boys			Females	Males	Females	Males	Females	Males
Vegetables and Fruit	4	5	6	7	8	7-8	8-10	7	7
Grain Products	3	4	6	6	7	6-7	8	6	7
Milk and Alternatives	2	2	3-4	3-4	3-4	2	2	3	3
Meat and Alternatives	1	1	1-2	2	3	2	3	2	3

What is One Food Guide Serving?
Look at the examples below.

Fresh, frozen or canned vegetables
125 mL (½ cup)

Bread
1 slice (35 g)

Bagel
½ bagel (45 g)

Milk or powdered milk (reconstituted)
250 mL (1 cup)

Cooked fish, shellfish, poultry, lean meat
75 g (2 ½ oz.)/125 mL (½ cup)

The chart above shows how many Food Guide Servings you need from each of the four food groups every day.

Having the amount and type of food recommended and following the tips in *Canada's Food Guide* will help:

- Meet your needs for vitamins, minerals and other nutrients.
- Reduce your risk of obesity, type 2 diabetes, heart disease, certain types of cancer and osteoporosis.
- Contribute to your overall health and vitality.

For a full guide, please contact Health Canada or visit their website.

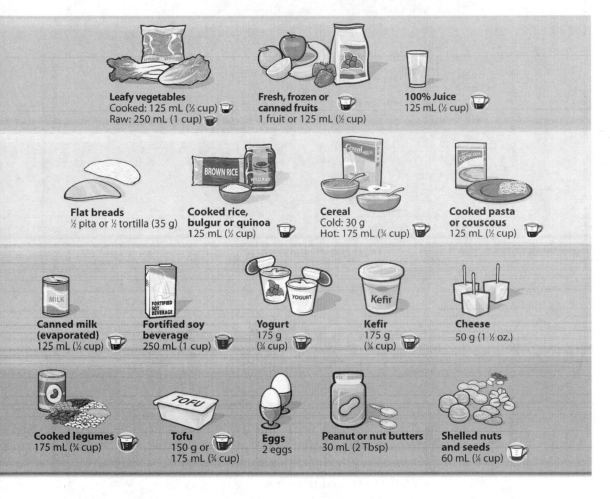

Leafy vegetables
Cooked: 125 mL (½ cup)
Raw: 250 mL (1 cup)

Fresh, frozen or canned fruits
1 fruit or 125 mL (½ cup)

100% Juice
125 mL (½ cup)

Flat breads
½ pita or ½ tortilla (35 g)

Cooked rice, bulgur or quinoa
125 mL (½ cup)

Cereal
Cold: 30 g
Hot: 175 mL (¾ cup)

Cooked pasta or couscous
125 mL (½ cup)

Canned milk (evaporated)
125 mL (½ cup)

Fortified soy beverage
250 mL (1 cup)

Yogurt
175 g
(¾ cup)

Kefir
175 g
(¾ cup)

Cheese
50 g (1 ½ oz.)

Cooked legumes
175 mL (¾ cup)

Tofu
150 g or
175 mL (¾ cup)

Eggs
2 eggs

Peanut or nut butters
30 mL (2 Tbsp)

Shelled nuts and seeds
60 mL (¼ cup)

Oils and Fats

- Include a small amount – 30 to 45 mL (2 to 3 Tbsp) – of unsaturated fat each day. This includes oil used for cooking, salad dressings, margarine and mayonnaise.
- Use vegetable oils such as canola, olive and soybean.
- Choose soft margarines that are low in saturated and trans fats.
- Limit butter, hard margarine, lard and shortening.

ChooseMyPlate.gov

Balancing Calories
- Enjoy your food, but eat less.
- Avoid oversized portions.

Foods to Increase
- Make half your plate fruits and vegetables.
- Make at least half your grains whole grains.
- Switch to fat-free or low-fat (1%) milk.

Foods to Reduce
- Compare sodium in foods like soup, bread, and frozen meals, and choose the foods with lower numbers.
- Drink water instead of sugary drinks.

Vegetarian food guide rainbow

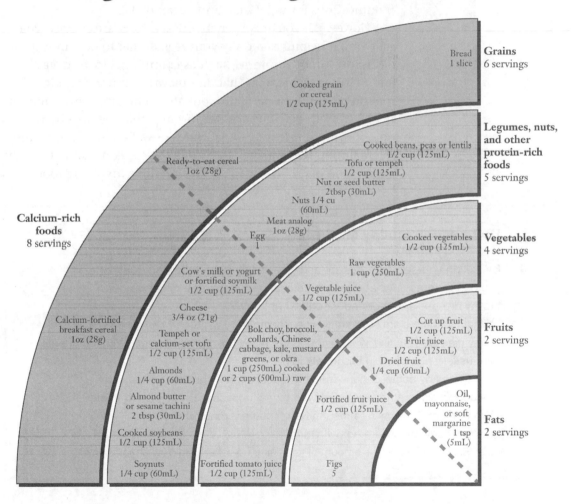

Grains
6 servings

Bread
1 slice

Cooked grain
or cereal
1/2 cup (125mL)

Ready-to-eat cereal
1oz (28g)

**Legumes, nuts,
and other
protein-rich
foods**
5 servings

Cooked beans, peas or lentils
1/2 cup (125mL)

Tofu or tempeh
1/2 cup (125mL)

Nut or seed butter
2tbsp (30mL)

Nuts 1/4 cu
(60mL)

Meat analog
1oz (28g)

Egg
1

**Calcium-rich
foods**
8 servings

Vegetables
4 servings

Cooked vegetables
1/2 cup (125mL)

Raw vegetables
1 cup (250mL)

Cow's milk or yogurt
or fortified soymilk
1/2 cup (125mL)

Vegetable juice
1/2 cup (125mL)

Cheese
3/4 oz (21g)

Calcium-fortified
breakfast cereal
1oz (28g)

Tempeh or
calcium-set tofu
1/2 cup (125mL)

Bok choy, broccoli,
collards, Chinese
cabbage, kale, mustard
greens, or okra
1 cup (250mL) cooked
or 2 cups (500mL) raw

Fruits
2 servings

Cut up fruit
1/2 cup (125mL)

Fruit juice
1/2 cup (125mL)

Dried fruit
1/4 cup (60mL)

Almonds
1/4 cup (60mL)

Almond butter
or sesame tachini
2 tbsp (30mL)

Fortified fruit juice
1/2 cup (125mL)

Oil,
mayonnaise,
or soft
margarine
1 tsp
(5mL)

Fats
2 servings

Cooked soybeans
1/2 cup (125mL)

Soynuts
1/4 cup (60mL)

Fortified tomato juice
1/2 cup (125mL)

Figs
5

Source: Figure 2 - A new food guide for North American vegetarians. Messina V, Melina V, Mangels AR. *Can Diet Pract Res.* 2003; 64 (2):82. Copyright 2003. Dietitians of Canada. Used with permission.

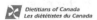

Dietitians of Canada
Les diététistes du Canada

Diet Modifications

If your IBD is under control and you live relatively symptom free, there is no need to restrict foods or follow a special diet. Just follow the United States Department of Agriculture (USDA) MyPlate Food Guidance System or Canada's Food Guide. The Dietitians of Canada have also created a Vegetarian Food Guide Rainbow. These reliable diet guides emphasize eating a wide variety of foods that provide the multitude of nutrients your body needs. The key is to select a variety of foods from all food groups in the recommended amounts, with appropriate modifications for vegetarian and vegan diets.

However, if you are experiencing acute disease activity, you may find it helpful to modify your regular diet to help minimize gastrointestinal symptoms, such as cramping, bloating, gas, and diarrhea. Remember that diet plays an important role in maintaining nutritional status, but also in helping with symptom management. It is of utmost importance that dietary changes do not compromise nutritional status or well-being. This means maintaining weight and energy-intake levels, continuing to enjoy eating, and participating in social situations involving food.

 Do I need to modify my diet?

 By asking yourself, your doctor, and your dietitian the following questions, you can determine what dietary modifications, if any, you might require:
- Is my disease active or under control right now?
- What symptoms am I currently experiencing?
- If my disease is active, what part or parts of my bowel are affected? What nutrients are usually absorbed in this location?
- Are there any complications from my disease that I should also consider — osteoporosis or strictures (narrowed bowel from scar tissue), for example?
- What effect does my treatment have on nutrient requirements?
- Do my medications interact with nutrients?
- Has surgery affected the amount of remaining bowel available for absorption?

Diet Modification Goals

There are specific goals for diet modifications to address not only symptom management, but also to help achieve better physical and emotional health. For instance, there can be a feeling of social isolation when your food choices are limited or you need to ask for special accommodations when eating away from home. Sometimes you just want to feel "normal" like everyone else.

Diet Modification Goals

1. **Normalize bowel function**
   - Decrease stool frequency
   - Increase stool consistency

2. **Minimize GI intolerance symptoms**
   - Reduce gas, bloating, cramping, pain
   - Reduce obstruction risk

3. **Maintain hydration and electrolyte balance**

4. **Maintain or improve nutritional status**
   - Prevent further weight loss (or weight gain if applicable)
   - Improve functional status
   - Supplement with specific nutrients if indicated

5. **Continue or resume social participation and enjoyment**
   - Normalize diet with time
   - Improve relationship with food

Elimination Diets

Elimination diets are popular in the diet industry, and complementary and alternative medicine practitioners may also take this approach to treatment. This type of diet significantly restricts or excludes one or more foods or major food groups. Common examples of exclusions include dairy, wheat or gluten, red meat, yeast, and refined sugars. If you choose to follow an elimination diet, be sure to consider the potential side effects.

Side Effects

Consequences of following exclusionary diets over the long term — that is, for more than a few weeks — include possible development of nutrient deficiencies, weight loss, malnutrition, food phobias or obsessions, and a loss of enjoyment of eating. If major food groups are avoided, be sure to speak with a dietitian to learn about alternative foods or supplements for the excluded nutrients.

Exclusion Diet Value

The value of exclusion diets has not been scientifically proven in IBD. In studies where suspected foods were excluded, individuals didn't experience disease relapse upon reintroduction of the excluded foods.

There is also a psychological danger with elimination diets. Following a diet that claims to control your IBD can contribute to a feeling of being somehow responsible or guilty if your disease becomes active again. Some people feel they may have cheated on the diet because they had difficulty following it exactly, and they are now responsible for their disease coming back. There is no evidence to support this. This type of internalization of responsibility is destructive and takes strength away during a time when it is difficult enough to live with IBD.

If you still feel it is important to try this approach, be sure to set a timeline for evaluating and stopping the dietary eliminations.

Lactose-Restricted Diets

Is there ever a time when it may be appropriate to reduce consumption or avoid a particular food group? When it comes to dairy products, the answer is yes. "Delicious but caution warranted" is a slogan to apply to dairy products if you have IBD. While dairy products are tasty and provide important nutrients, such as protein and calcium, there are specific situations where it may be difficult to digest the primary sugar in milk.

Unless you have a true milk allergy (immune reaction to the protein in milk), there is no danger from eating dairy products. This type of allergy is relatively uncommon. Dairy products do not cause IBD and generally do not result in flares, but you may experience uncomfortable symptoms if you have lactose intolerance and you drink milk or eat dairy products.

Lactase Deficiency

Lactose is the principal carbohydrate in dairy products. It is a disaccharide, meaning that it is a larger molecule made up of two smaller sugar molecules, which are the monosaccharides glucose and galactose. An enzyme called lactase in our small intestine is responsible for breaking lactose into glucose and galactose, which are then easily absorbed.

If there is not enough lactase enzyme available to break down lactose into its two smaller sugars, the result is undigested lactose traveling through the small intestine to the large intestine (colon). This is why lactose intolerance can also be correctly called lactase deficiency.

Lactose Intolerance Symptoms

The classic symptoms of lactose intolerance result from undigested lactose traveling through the small bowel and drawing water by osmosis into the bowel, which causes bloating. When the undigested lactose reaches the colon, bacteria ferment it, producing further bloating, cramping, gas, and diarrhea. Symptoms vary among individuals, but typically appear within 30 minutes to several hours after ingestion.

 How do I know if I might be susceptible to lactose intolerance?

 There are at least two possible factors involved in causing lactose intolerance: genetics and acquired factors.

Genetics: The most common cause of lactose intolerance in adults has to do with genetics. There is a natural decline in lactase production as we age (genetically determined rate). This natural decline in the amount of lactase enzyme present on the surface of the small bowel occurs as people age and leads to progressive lactose intolerance (this is called primary lactase deficiency).

Although everyone experiences a decrease in lactase production over their lifetime, the rate at which this occurs is different for different ethnic groups. Certain ethnic groups have a genetic predisposition to lactase deficiency, including individuals of African, Jewish, and Asian descent. Conversely, individuals of Scandinavian and Northern European descent have the lowest prevalence of lactose intolerance. North Americans of similar ancestry have demonstrated similar prevalence rates.

Acquired Lactase Deficiency: External factors can sometimes result in a deficiency in the amount of lactase enzyme available on the small bowel surface (called secondary lactase deficiency). This may occur following medical treatment (for example, chemotherapy, radiation, or multiple small bowel resections), in malnutrition, or from active small intestinal disease, such as Crohn's disease. Once the disease or injury resolves, lactase production resumes and digestion of lactose usually improves, but not always.

Lactose Intolerance Testing

A hydrogen breath test, which involves drinking a test dose of lactose, can help to determine if you are lactose intolerant. If a person has lactase deficiency, the unabsorbed lactose will be fermented by colonic bacteria and hydrogen gas will be formed. Some of this hydrogen gas is absorbed into your bloodstream and breathed out through the lungs, where it can be measured in your breath.

If you have a hydrogen breath test, be sure to ask what dose of lactose you were tested with. Depending on the lab, doses can range anywhere from 12.5 g of lactose (equivalent to 1 cup/250 mL of milk) to 50 g of lactose (equivalent to 4 cups/1 L of milk). Many people can drink one glass of milk without difficulty, but would rarely drink a quart or liter of milk at one time, so the relevance (applicability to your daily life) of the test depends on the dose administered.

Dairy Reduction

Fortunately, many individuals who develop lactose intolerance can still consume small amounts of dairy, just not as much as before. This is called a dose-dependent effect. In these cases, eliminating dairy products is not necessary, just a reduction in the amount of dairy product taken at one time. Interestingly, some people can gradually increase their tolerance to dairy. This has nothing to do with the amount of lactase enzyme they have, but rather their gastrointestinal bacteria are able to adapt to the lactose load.

Lactose Ladder

This lactose ladder lists dairy products and their lactose content. You can start climbing from the bottom (lowest lactose-containing foods) and make your way as far up to the top (higher lactose-containing foods) as you can tolerate.

Source	Serving	Lactose (grams)
Milk (homogenized 3.25%, 2%, 1%, skim)	1 cup (250 mL)	12.0–13.0
Yogurt (with probiotics to reduce lactose)	½ cup (125 mL)	6.3-9.5
Ice cream	½ cup (125 mL)	4.9
Frozen yogurt	½ cup (125 mL)	4.5
Cottage cheese	½ cup (125 mL)	2.9–3.9
Sour cream	¼ cup (60 mL)	2.0
Cream cheese	1 oz (30 g)	0.7
Cream (heavy or whipping, half-and-half)	1 tbsp (15 mL)	0.6
Cheese (Cheddar, Gouda, blue, Colby)	1 oz (30 g)	0.5–0.8
Dry curd cottage cheese	½ cup (125 mL)	0.5
Parmesan cheese	1 tbsp (15 mL), grated	0.2
Cheese (Camembert, Limburger)	1 oz (30 g)	0.1
Butter	1 tsp (5 mL)	Trace

Hidden Lactose

There are also hidden sources of lactose in foods. If you are severely lactose intolerant, you will need to avoid all sources of lactose. Lactose can be added as a filler in some medications and some foods (for example, processed meats, gravies, breads, cereals, salad dressings, breakfast drinks, cake mixes, margarine). Lactose may also be present if the label lists added milk solids, whey, curds, butter, or cheese flavor. Casein does not contain lactose. Be sure to read food labels for hidden sources.

 Q **Should I try reducing or avoiding lactose?**

 A Controversy exists regarding the clinical prevalence of secondary lactase deficiency in IBD. This is because the lactose intolerance studies have not always taken age or ethnicity into account (factors we know affect the amount of lactase enzyme). Lactose intolerance may be more common in IBD; however, this is not definitive. Often doctors will ask a person to restrict dairy in the diet temporarily to determine how the disease is responding to treatment and to prevent misdiagnosis of any lactose intolerance symptoms as disease activity symptoms. Bloating, cramping, and diarrhea could be misdiagnosed as ongoing IBD symptoms.

If your symptoms improve while avoiding lactose, then a temporary restriction is right for you. If not, it is important not to restrict dairy from your diet unnecessarily. When your flare improves, it is worthwhile increasing dairy in your diet again. This is especially true if you tolerated dairy products before your flare or if you miss eating dairy products.

Ileostomy

If you have an ileostomy and are lactose intolerant, you can still eat dairy products. The undigested lactose will reach the ileostomy pouch instead of being fermented in the colon (which may have been surgically removed). The ileostomy pouch may develop more gas (from the bacteria in the stool), but it will not give you the same symptoms of cramping, bloating, and diarrhea.

Calcium Sources

Dairy products are important sources of calcium, and some of these products are fortified with vitamin D. Calcium and vitamin D are critical for good bone and tooth health (other important nutrients for bone health include phosphorus, magnesium, and fluoride). A diet that includes adequate amounts of these nutrients is one important factor to help prevent bone loss (osteopenia) and development of osteoporosis.

Other Food Sources of Calcium

You may limit dairy because of lactose intolerance or avoid it entirely for other reasons, such as taste, ethics, allergy, or cultural or religious traditions. Regardless of the reason, the challenge is to get the key nutrients provided by this food group in other ways. Calcium from dairy products is better absorbed than calcium from many other foods.

Enzyme Supplements

Another strategy for consuming adequate calcium when you are lactose intolerant is to use a commercial lactase enzyme product to break down lactose. These are available as tablets or as liquid drops in most pharmacies.

Q Am I getting enough calcium?

A Recommended amounts (known as Dietary Reference Intakes, or DRIs) for nutrients are based on age and gender. In adults, the range for calcium is generally 1000 to 1300 mg per day, depending on your age, gender, if you are pregnant, if you have osteoporosis, or if you have any condition that affects metabolism or absorption of calcium and vitamin D (check with your health-care team to find the specific amount recommended for you). In clinical practice, doctors advise amounts that also take bone health and medication use (for example, steroid use) into consideration.

Lactose-free products (milk, yogurt, ice cream) will contain the same amount of calcium (and the same amount of vitamin D, in the case of milk and some yogurts) as their lactose-containing versions (only the lactose content has changed). The absorption of calcium from plant-based sources is reduced due to compounds called oxalates (found in dark green leafy vegetables, such as spinach and beet greens) and phytates (found in whole grains, nuts, seeds, and legumes). These foods have decreased bioavailability of calcium because the oxalates and phytates bind to minerals, such as calcium, thus interfering with absorption.

If you suspect you are not meeting the recommended amounts for calcium or vitamin D, consult with your doctor or a registered dietitian.

Dairy Sources of Calcium

In order to get enough calcium, it is recommended that adults consume two to four servings of milk products per day. This table lists common lactose-containing sources of calcium (milligrams of calcium rounded) approximated to usual serving sizes.

Source	Serving	Calcium (mg)
Cow's milk (skim, 1%, 2%, whole, chocolate, buttermilk) and goat's milk	1 cup (250 mL)	285–330
Evaporated milk, partly skimmed	½ cup (125 mL)	350
Powdered milk	6 tbsp (90 mL), dry	320
Milk kefir	¾ cup (175 mL)	187–198
Cream soup (made with milk)	1 cup (250 mL)	175–190
Pudding (made with milk)	½ cup (125 mL)	105–165
Yogurt (plain or flavored or fruit bottom)	¾ cup (175 mL)	215–325
Yogurt drink	¾ cup (175 mL)	185
Frozen yogurt	½ cup (125 mL)	150
Ice cream or ice milk	½ cup (125 mL)	80–90
Sour cream (nonfat)	½ cup (125 mL)	225
Cottage cheese (1% or 2%)	½ cup (125 mL)	70–85
Processed cheese: thin slice thick slice	2 slices (1½ oz/42 g) 2 slices (2 oz/62 g)	255 385
Cheese (soft) • Brie • Camembert • Ricotta (part skim) Cheese (hard) • Parmesan cheese • Cheddar, Gouda, Colby, Edam, brick, Swiss cheese • Feta cheese • Mozzarella	 1¾ oz (50 g) 1¾ oz (50 g) ½ cup (125 mL) 3 tbsp (45 mL), grated 1¾ oz (50 g) 1¾ oz (50 g) 1¾ oz (50 g)	 90 195 340 260 350–480 255 270

Supplements

If you don't think you can improve your intake from food and beverages, consider calcium supplements with vitamin D and discuss this with your doctor. There may be times when your doctor recommends supplements in addition to foods. There are many forms of calcium supplements to choose from — pills, effervescent tablets, chewable tablets, and "soft chews" in multiple flavors. Be sure to choose calcium supplements that also contain vitamin D.

Alternative Food Sources of Calcium

Consider the following suggestions for alternative food and supplement sources of calcium (milligrams of calcium rounded).

Source	Serving	Calcium (mg)
Fortified soy milk (absorption of calcium may be slightly less than cow's milk)	1 cup (250 mL)	300
Fortified orange juice	$\frac{1}{2}$ cup (125 mL)	150
Fortified apple juice	1 cup (250 mL)	92
Orange	1 (medium)	50
Fortified rice beverage	1 cup (250 mL)	300
Fortified plant-based beverages — almond, hemp, coconut, cashew "milk" (nut beverages do not contain the same nutrients as cow's milk or soy milk; for example, they contain less protein)	1 cup (250 mL)	Varies (check label)
Tofu (soft) set with calcium sulphate	$\frac{1}{3}$ cup (75 mL)	150 (check label)
Nuts and seeds • Almonds • Brazil nuts (dried) • Sesame seeds (whole dried)	 1 oz (30 g), 24 nuts 1 oz (30 g), 8 medium nuts 1 tbsp (15 mL)	 75 50 88
Legumes (cooked) • Baked or refried beans • Chickpeas • Red kidney beans • Navy, white, soybeans	 1 cup (250 mL) 1 cup (250 mL) 1 cup (250 mL) 1 cup (250 mL)	 130–165 85 50 90–200
Vegetables (cooked) • Spinach • Broccoli • Bok choy, kale, Swiss chard • Collard greens	 $\frac{1}{2}$ cup (125 mL) $\frac{1}{2}$ cup (125 mL) $\frac{1}{2}$ cup (125 mL) $\frac{1}{2}$ cup (125 mL)	 130 40–50 50–105 180
Pink or sockeye salmon (with bones)	$\frac{1}{2}$ can ($\frac{2}{3}$ cup/175 mL)	225–240
Sardines (with bones)	$\frac{1}{2}$ can (2 oz/55 g), 4 pieces	200
Blackstrap molasses	1 tsp (5 mL)	60
Figs (dried)	6	150

Optimal Dose

On the label, look at the "elemental" calcium content — that is, the calcium available to your body. Split calcium dosages so that you are taking no more than 500 mg elemental calcium at any one time in order to get maximal absorption. For some forms of calcium, take the supplements with meals. Calcium carbonate, for example, requires stomach acid for absorption, whereas calcium citrate or gluconate do not.

Discuss the safest sources of calcium supplements with your pharmacist. Dolomite or bone meal, for example, are most contaminated by lead; oyster shell or shellfish sources may pass government standards; and calcium citrate and refined calcium carbonates are considered lowest in lead content.

Vitamin D

Vitamin D helps your body absorb calcium. Interestingly, vitamin D is a hormone that our bodies make when sunlight shines on our skin (sunlight provides ultraviolet radiation for the body to convert vitamin D to an active form). In northern latitudes of North America and Europe, the reduced sunshine and angle of the sun in winter months results in less vitamin D manufactured by the skin. Similarly, if individuals have dark skin (more pigmentation), are housebound or institutionalized, or wear sunscreen at all times when outdoors, they are also at risk of not getting enough vitamin D. Generally speaking, if you have between 5 and 30 minutes of sunlight exposure between 10 a.m. and 3 p.m. (face, arms, hands, without sunscreen) twice a week, you are probably getting enough vitamin D. What can influence this estimate is your geographic location, the time of year, your age, and your skin color.

Fortified?

Milk is almost always fortified with vitamin D, but not all dairy products are good sources of vitamin D. For instance, cottage cheese is not made from fortified milk, so it does not provide much vitamin D. Some food manufacturers are starting to add vitamin D to some products, so just check the label.

Optimal Dose

Because of the factors that interfere with our ability to get enough vitamin D, select items in our food supply are fortified with vitamin D. The combination of sun exposure, food sources, and supplements is thought to allow most North Americans to meet their vitamin D needs. The importance of vitamin D relates to its well-established positive role with respect to building and maintaining bone health. Vitamin D has also recently been evaluated for its purported benefit of protecting against other chronic diseases, including cancer, cardiovascular disease, and diabetes. However, there has been insufficient evidence to date that a higher intake will confer these benefits.

In 2010, the Food and Nutrition Board at the Institute of Medicine (IOM), which is the health arm of the National Academy of Sciences, published revised recommendations for the recommended amount of vitamin D intake. In its report, commissioned by the American and Canadian governments, the DRI for vitamin D for adults was raised from 200 IU to 600 to

Vitamin D Sources

Source	Serving	Vitamin D (IU)
Cow's milk	1 cup (250 mL)	90–100
Fortified soy milk or plant-based beverage	1 cup (250 mL)	90–100 (check label)
Fortified yogurt	¾ cup (175 mL)	88 (check label)
Fortified orange juice	1 cup (250 mL)	100
Fortified margarine	1 tbsp (15 mL)	60
Salmon	3 oz (90 g), cooked	360–500
Mackerel	3 oz (90 g), cooked	388
Sardines	1¾ oz (50 g), canned	250
Tuna	3 oz (90 g), canned	200
Egg	1 yolk	20–25
Cod liver oil (avoid this source because it may contain contaminants, as well as high levels of vitamin A, which can weaken bones)	1 tbsp (15 mL)	1400

Note: Be sure to check whether the fortification is with the preferred form of vitamin D_3 and not vitamin D_2, which is less potent.

800 IU, depending on age and sex (for example, a higher amount is recommended for high-risk groups such as the elderly). There has been considerable discussion following the publication of these guidelines, and some public health organizations (for example, the Canadian Cancer Society, Canadian Pediatrics Society, and Osteoporosis Canada) have maintained recommendations for increased doses of vitamin D anywhere from 800 to 2000 IU per day.

Adults on prednisone may be advised to take 1500 mg of elemental calcium a day and 2000 IU of vitamin D. Vitamin D above these amounts can lead to significant health problems, so it is important to discuss any supplementation with your physician.

Other Vitamin and Mineral Supplements

Replacing or supplementing nutrients other than calcium and vitamin D may be necessary if there is a problem with absorption. Absorption of nutrients can be affected by disease activity, bacterial overgrowth, loss of bowel from surgical resections, or interference from medications.

Key micronutrients

Water-soluble vitamins	Fat-soluble vitamins	Minerals	Trace elements
• Vitamin B_1 (thiamin) • Vitamin B_2 (riboflavin) • Vitamin B_3 (niacin) • Pantothenic acid • Vitamin B_6 (pyridoxine) • Biotin • Folic acid • Vitamin B_{12} (cyanocobalamin) • Vitamin C	• Vitamin A (beta-carotene is the precursor) • Vitamin D • Vitamin E • Vitamin K	• Calcium • Chloride • Magnesium • Phosphorus • Potassium • Sodium • Sulphur	• Chromium • Copper • Fluoride • Iodine • Iron • Manganese • Molybdenum • Selenium • Zinc

Nutrient Deficiency Symptoms and Supplements

Calories: In general, if you are underweight and are not able to maintain a healthy weight, you may need to boost calories (calories come from macronutrients, namely carbohydrates, protein, and fat).

Protein: You may need extra protein if you are on high-dose steroids, extra protein and iron if you have ongoing blood loss, or additional protein and zinc if you have prolonged diarrhea, a wound, or a fistula affecting your small bowel.

Fat: You may need to change the amount and supplement a specific type of fat if you have extensive Crohn's disease of the ileum or have had more than 3 feet (1 m) of terminal ileum removed surgically.

Iron: If you have anemia, you might require supplementation of iron, folate, or vitamin B_{12}.

Vitamin B_{12}: You will most likely also need to replace vitamin B_{12} by injection or by tablets dissolved under the tongue if your disease is active in your terminal ileum or you have had large amounts of terminal ileum surgically resected at one or more operations.

Folic acid: If you are taking sulfasalazine or methotrexate, you will likely need to supplement folate, as these drugs interfere with folate's metabolism. Note that folic acid is the correct term for a supplement of folate.

Sodium and Potassium: If you have had your large bowel removed or have persistent watery diarrhea, you will likely need to increase fluid and electrolytes (sodium and potassium) in your diet.

Calcium and Vitamin D: If you are treated with steroids, you will probably need additional calcium and vitamin D because steroids interfere with the absorption of calcium. Another medication called cholestyramine interferes with the absorption of fat-soluble vitamins, such as vitamin D.

Vitamin B12 Injections

Vitamin B12 is absorbed only in the terminal ileum (the last part of the small intestine), so if you have Crohn's disease in that region or have had surgical resection of your terminal ileum, you most likely require supplements. Vitamin B12 absorption is also dependent on intrinsic factor (IF), which is secreted by the stomach, so people who have had surgery to remove part of the stomach may also require vitamin B12 supplements. Because the terminal ileum is diseased or removed, vitamin B12 won't be absorbed if you take a supplement by mouth — it must be delivered by injection. (In some cases, vitamin B12 injections can be replaced with vitamin B12 pills that dissolve under the tongue and are absorbed more easily.)

Frequently Asked Questions about Vitamin and Mineral Supplements

If you think you may need to supplement specific nutrients, talk to your doctor.

 Should I take a multivitamin supplement?

 Supplements are a good idea when a major food group is eliminated. But what about taking a supplement for times when you are busy and you do not necessarily take the time to plan, shop for, prepare, or eat nutritious meals? These regular daily activities can be especially hard for someone who isn't feeling well or is lacking in energy.

The best way to determine whether you need a supplement is to identify which food groups are not well represented in your daily diet. Remember, vitamins, minerals, and trace elements are essential to your health because your body cannot synthesize them. They must be consumed from a variety of foods.

The first step is to compare your diet to the USDA MyPlate Food Guidance System or Canada's Food Guide. For each food, a particular set of nutrients and a recommended number of servings are specified. For example, the grain products are significant sources of complex carbohydrates, riboflavin, thiamin, niacin, iron, protein, magnesium, and fiber. Thus, if an individual does not choose many servings from this group, those nutrients may be lacking. This is when it is a good idea to consider a supplement for the missing nutrients. Just remember that eating the real thing is more tasty, filling, and provides more nutrient variety. A well-balanced diet, including a variety of foods, is best for good health and can usually be eaten even if you have IBD.

Q What vitamin and mineral supplements should I take?

A There are many brands of standard adult multivitamins with minerals, and most varieties are fine for meeting general needs. There are special versions available, which add more target nutrients (for example, prenatal versions have more iron, calcium, and folic acid, while "silver" versions add more calcium for people over 50 years old).

More does not necessarily mean better. The "mega" or "super" or "stress" doses are not usually more beneficial because any excess that is ingested is not used by your body and is simply excreted in the urine or stored in the liver or fat tissue, which can be harmful.

There are safety risks to mega-dosing, especially with fat-soluble vitamins, which are stored in our bodies and not excreted in urine. Harm from higher doses can include toxicities; masking deficiencies of other nutrients (for example, folic acid masks vitamin B_{12} deficiency); interference with body functions, such as blood clotting (for example, excess vitamin E); risk of birth defects; liver damage (for example, excess vitamin A); or risk of kidney stones (for example, excess calcium).

Q Are vitamins and mineral supplements safe?

A In addition to considering the appropriate dose, how do you know if the product is safe?

In the United States, vitamins and minerals (as well as botanical products and herbs) are considered "dietary supplements" under the Dietary Supplement Health and Education Act (DSHEA) of 1994. According to this act, a company is responsible for determining that the dietary supplements it makes or distributes are safe. They must also have evidence for any claims of health benefits, but they do not need approval from the Food and Drug Administration (FDA) before they market the product. The manufacturer is responsible for listing the ingredients of the supplements, but the FDA does not monitor the quality of the dietary supplements on a routine basis. Manufacturers who introduce new supplements after 1994 are required to show evidence of the safety of their product.

In Canada, when choosing a supplement, look for a D.I.N. (drug identification number) or a G.P. (general product) number, which assures you that Health Canada has approved the product as safe. This way, you know that you are getting what you are paying for. Products with a D.I.N. undergo quality assurance testing to ensure standardization, safety, and effectiveness.

What about herbs?

 In the United States, botanical and herbal products are considered to be "dietary supplements," similar to the situation with vitamins and minerals, and manufacturers are responsible for ensuring the safety and content of their products.

In Canada, botanical and herbal products are considered natural and nonprescription health products (NNHPs) and do not have D.I.N.s. Regulation of NNHPs is in progress, and an advisory committee appointed by Health Canada, called the Natural and Nonprescription Health Products Directorate (NNHPD), is supervising clinical trials of products. This is a costly process for the companies that manufacture and market NNHPs, but it is important for consumers to ensure each NNHP will contain the stated amount of active ingredient and that it is safe (from contaminants, for example) and effective. This process of regulation came into place in 2004.

Liquid Calorie Supplements

During times when you feel that you cannot get enough calories, you may want to drink commercially prepared liquid supplements. There are many different brand names, varieties, and flavors. Most are lactose free.

Kinds of Liquid Supplements

There are several different kinds of liquid supplements designed for specific purposes. Consult with your doctor or dietitian before choosing one.

Polymeric

Standard versions of oral supplements are called polymeric because the carbohydrates, fats, and protein molecules are provided as complete undigested molecules. This is the way we would find them in food. Other products are designed to help with impaired digestion.

Semi-Elemental

In semi-elemental products, the protein has been broken down (hydrolyzed) into smaller molecules. These smaller components of proteins are called peptides, and these can be made of two, three, or several amino acids joined together (amino acids are the most basic building block of protein).

Elemental

Another specialized type of supplement is called elemental because the protein is hydrolyzed into its most basic components (free amino acids). These supplements usually contain fats and carbohydrates in partially digested (simplest forms) as well.

These products are designed to be more easily absorbed when digestion is impaired. For this reason, they usually contain medium-chain triglycerides (MCTs) as part of their fat content. MCTs do not require digestion and can be absorbed directly from the gut. The amount of fat in these specialized medical foods may also be reduced. The manufacturing companies are also starting to include more healthy fat sources, such as canola oil (to increase the amount of anti-inflammatory omega-3 fat) instead of corn oil (thus reducing the pro-inflammatory omega-6 fat content).

Modular

You may also wish to supplement just one specific nutrient. Medical products designed to do this are called modular supplements. Examples include Polycose (carbohydrate only), MCT oil (fat only), or protein powders. These can be added to many foods (easily added to liquids or moist foods).

Calorie- and Protein-Boosting Drinks

These can be made with cow's milk, soy beverage, or fruit beverages with added protein. Examples include Scandishake, which can provide close to 600 calories when made with 1 cup (250 mL) of whole milk, and Carnation Breakfast Essentials, which boosts calories and protein (but does contain lactose).

Primary Therapy

For Crohn's disease affecting the small bowel, nutritional supplements can be used as primary therapy to treat the inflammation and thereby reduce symptoms. This is not the case for ulcerative colitis. When individuals drink only supplements (or receive supplements via a feeding tube), they often find their disease goes into remission and they can avoid steroid medications. This is especially important for children and adolescents who want to avoid the negative side effects of steroids, such as delayed growth. Polymeric, semi-elemental, or elemental supplements all provide a beneficial effect.

Different theories have been proposed to account for the effectiveness of these supplements in some patients. The low number of microbes in the supplements compared to a regular diet, the beneficial effects of specific types of fat, and the beneficial effect of simply improving overall nutritional status, with a consequent improvement in immunity, may account for the effectiveness of supplements.

> **Full Requirements**
>
> Most liquid supplements have vitamins, minerals, and trace elements added. In order to meet the full requirements for these, a specific volume must be consumed. For an average person, you might need to drink four or five units (cans, boxes, Tetra Paks, or packages dissolved in water) every day in order to meet your needs.

Tips for Taking Supplements

- Discuss your supplements with your pharmacist because they are experts.
- Take fiber supplements separately because fiber may bind to some nutrients, thus interfering with their absorption.
- If supplementing fat-soluble vitamins, take with a meal because they require some fat to be better absorbed.
- If you require calcium supplements, take them separately from multivitamins because the iron in the multivitamin interferes with calcium absorption.
- Take medications cold (keep the container on ice) to ease swallowing.
- Mix supplements in water, cover, and sip with a straw to avoid the medicine odor.
- Flavor nutrition drinks with vanilla, mint, or banana extracts or flavor packets.
- Include in a milkshake or smoothie recipe.
- Substitute nutrition drinks for milk in baking recipes.

Low-Fiber Diets

Insoluble and Soluble Fiber

Both insoluble and soluble fiber are good for you, but if you are looking to reduce bowel movement frequency and thicken stool consistency, then you will probably want to increase your intake of soluble fiber. Likewise, to avoid increasing the frequency of bowel movements (such as during a disease flare), limit sources of insoluble fiber.

Dietitians and physicians usually recommend increasing fiber in your diet for overall good health. Fiber is important for weight management. Fiber may help manage blood sugar in diabetes, it may help manage diverticulosis, it may help reduce cholesterol, and it may help protect against some kinds of cancers. While eating fiber, you feel full sooner and may eat less. Despite these clear health benefits, your doctor or dietitian may ask you to limit fiber in your diet because you have IBD. The priority when you have an IBD flare is to recover, return to better health, and have improved quality of life. This may require adjusting or reducing your fiber intake.

In clinical practice, a low-residue diet limits foods that increase the amount of undigested food matter and the amount of stool produced. The definition of low residue is not well supported by evidence, and as such, clinicians now refer to a low-fiber diet. Low-fiber diets allow soluble fiber, but limit insoluble fiber and foods that could potentially contribute to food-related obstructions.

This fiber-restricted diet is intended to be only a short-term diet to help you feel more comfortable by decreasing gastrointestinal intolerance symptoms from a flare or from a change in the normal anatomy after surgery. This is not a fiber-free diet; rather, there is a compromise by allowing

Q **What is fiber?**

A Fiber is the structural part of plants (vegetables, fruits, grains, and legumes). Human digestive enzymes cannot break down fiber; however, some bacteria in the gastrointestinal tract can break it down. Dietary fiber can be fermented by colonic bacteria to produce short-chain fatty acids (SCFA), which are absorbed and provide the body with energy (used specifically by the cells that line your intestine and liver).

Fiber is commonly classified according to its solubility (ability to dissolve in fluid) as insoluble or soluble. Insoluble fiber is not easily fermented by bacteria and is best known for bulking stool and relieving constipation. It increases the fecal weight and speeds up the passage of material through the intestines. Soluble fiber is fermented by many bacteria in the large intestine and is best known for its favorable effects on cholesterol. It also slows stomach emptying and passage of material through the intestines, helping to form or gel loose bowel movements. Both kinds of fiber slow starch breakdown, thus slowing glucose absorption into the bloodstream; both create a full feeling; and both contribute to gas production (and thus need to be introduced and increased gradually in the diet.)

soluble fiber until you can comfortably include sources of insoluble fibre in your diet again. The goal is for you to return to a regular diet once your disease and symptoms have improved. In the meantime, be sure to plan meals in advance so that you can find acceptable alternatives and have them available to you when you are hungry.

Long-Term Low-Fiber Diet

There are times when a low-fiber diet needs to be followed over a longer period of time. Such is the case when you have narrowing of the bowel due to scar tissue or stricturing of the intestine in Crohn's disease. When there is narrowing, the bowels must push hard to pass undigested food matter through the narrowed area. This causes cramping, pain, and, in some cases, abdominal bloating and nausea.

Similar situations of bowel narrowing occur with inflammation from active Crohn's disease and bowel-wall swelling following surgery. This is usually temporary because the swelling decreases with treatment or time and the size of the opening of the bowel returns to normal. Unfortunately, scar tissue remains despite treatment with medication. In that case, the narrowing is permanent, unless it is surgically removed or corrected.

Cocktail Caution

Beware of so-called juice cocktails, because they contain only a small amount of natural fruit juice, while the rest is water with large amounts of sugar in the form of high-fructose corn syrup, dextrose, or sugar/glucose-fructose. Look for the label "100% fruit juice" or "100% juice blends." Natural juice provides more vitamins, minerals, trace elements, and natural antioxidants than juice cocktails.

Long-term compliance with a low-fiber diet brings unique challenges for ensuring that vitamins, minerals, and trace elements are adequate, considering the many restrictions to the fruits and vegetables food group. The key is to rely on fruits and vegetables that are canned, well cooked, squeezed into juices, or puréed and strained. Sometimes a multivitamin and mineral supplement is needed, and these are now available for adults in chewable and "gummy" forms.

Fiber Fortification

To include more soluble fiber in your diet, try adding oat bran to moist foods, such as yogurt, pudding, sauces, and soups, as well as in baked goods (muffins or cookies) and cereal. You can even sprinkle oat bran onto your oatmeal! Try adding chickpeas or lentils to a casserole, or include kidney beans in a stew (but make sure to peel off and discard the outer skin). You can substitute applesauce for oil in a muffin recipe (also lower fat!). Add barley to soup, or make split pea soup. Slice bananas into Jell-O or yogurt for dessert.

Fiber Sources

Insoluble Fiber	Soluble Fiber
• Skins of fruits and vegetables (skins of peppers, eggplant, tomato, corn, apple) • Seeds of fruits and vegetables (kiwi, oranges, eggplant, field cucumbers, tomato) • Membranes of fruits and vegetables (sections of oranges, grapefruit) • Whole wheat and whole-grain breads and cereals • Brown or wild rice • White whole wheat flour (contains the bran and germ and thus the same fiber as whole wheat but looks like refined flour)	• Oat products: oatmeal and oat bran (breads, muffins, cookies, hot or cold cereals) • Barley • Tapioca • Psyllium fiber (powder, biscuit, or capsule, including Metamucil, Prodiem, or generic house brands) • Methylcellulose (Citrucel) • Pectin • Banana flakes • Pulp of fruits (flesh of orange, apple, grapefruit, banana) • Vegetables (okra) • Legumes (chickpeas, kidney beans, lentils with outer skin peeled)

Food Label Caution

It is important to read labels when choosing products for fiber content. For example, if a food product lists bran as a component, it most likely is wheat bran, a source of insoluble fiber; however, if the product specifies "oat" in front of "bran," as in "oat bran," it is a source of soluble fiber.

Kellogg's All-Bran Buds cereal with psyllium, for example, advertises one of the highest sources of fiber per serving. The label also lists "psyllium seed husk," which would lead one to think the cereal is a high source of psyllium and thus soluble fiber. Soluble fiber is good, right? The problem is that while each serving packs 3 g of soluble fiber, it also packs a whopping 9.7 g of insoluble fiber. If you read the ingredient list, wheat bran is the first listed ingredient, meaning that it constitutes the largest proportion of ingredients in the product. As a source of insoluble fiber, wheat bran will promote the opposite effect that you are looking for from the small soluble fiber content!

High-Stool-Output Management Diets

Sometimes modifying fiber isn't enough to slow down bowel movements. This can be the case during a flare or following multiple bowel resections if you have a high-output stoma or a pelvic pouch for ulcerative colitis. It is then appropriate to try some other diet strategies, provided you are receiving appropriate medical treatment for your condition.

There are many diet strategies that can be explored to help slow stool frequency and increase stool consistency. When making changes, try only one strategy at a time and for a few days. This way, if there is any benefit, you know what diet change is responsible. Conversely, you may find that you experience no positive effect, and you can then resume your usual intake and try other tips that might be helpful. Be sure to consult with your doctor or dietitians while trying these strategies.

Dietary Strategies to Slow High Stool Output

Modification	Explanation and Examples
• Increase soluble fiber	• Some people experience the most benefit from including soluble fiber at mealtime (not in between meals).
• Include foods known to thicken stool	• Cheese and cheesecake, smooth nut butters (peanut butter, almond butter, cashew butter), pretzels, potato chips, white rice (especially sticky rice like Arborio), tapioca, unleavened bread products (matzo and water crackers), gelatin-containing foods (Jell-O and marshmallows).
• Reduce dairy lactose	• If you reduce or eliminate dairy lactose, be sure to eat alternative calcium sources. • Try commercial lactase enzyme products.
• Reduce fat	• For extensive ileal Crohn's disease or ileal resection of more than 3 feet (1 m). This loss of bowel disrupts absorption of fat, and there is a greater loss of bile salts (normally reabsorbed in the ileum). • Try supplementing with MCT oil (available in specialty food shops), which is easily added to soups, beverages, salad dressings.
• Reduce simple sugars	• Sweets (jams, jellies, honey, maple syrup) and sweetened beverages (iced tea, fruit drinks, pop, soda, sports drinks, chocolate milk). • Sweetened plant-based milks (such as almond or soy milk), iced coffee drinks, sweetened coconut water. • Dilute concentrated sugar sources, such as fruit juices, and sip slowly.
• Reduce fructose	• A monosaccharide found naturally in fruits, but also a component of high-fructose corn syrup added to fruit drinks, soft drinks, baked goods, such as cookies. • Can cause an osmotic diarrhea at higher intakes (tolerance level is different for different people). • Fermented in colon by bacteria, thus contributing to gas.
• Reduce sugar alcohols	• Nutritive sweeteners that have about half the calories of regular sugar. Examples include sorbitol, mannitol, xylitol, and hydrogenated starch hydrolysates. • Found in hard candies, gum, mints, jams, and jellies. • Poorly absorbed and fermented in colon, contributing to gas, cramping, bloating, and diarrhea.
• Try gas-reducing strategies	• Gas is produced when fiber and residue from complex carbohydrates reach the colon. • Plan regular snacks between meals to reduce gas production (keep canned fruit with peel-back lids, granola bars, or individually wrapped oat bran cookies in your car's glove compartment or in a desk drawer at work).

Modification	Explanation and Examples
• Try gas-reducing strategies (continued)	• If consuming carbonated beverages, pour into a glass first and let stand for 10–15 minutes to reduce the carbonation. • Try commercial enzyme products (e.g., Beano, Phazyme), which predigest fiber and residue without forming gas. • Avoid smoking, chewing gum, using straws. • Chew foods well.
• Reduce caffeine and eliminate guarana	• Caffeine sources include coffee, tea (including green tea), hot chocolate, soft drinks (including dark colas and Mountain Dew). • Guarana comes from a shrub in the rainforest (seeds from its fruit are crushed, and these contain caffeine and other xanthines that stimulate bowel peristalsis). Examples of drinks with guarana include some varieties of beer and energy drinks. Avoid beer with added caffeine.
• Reduce alcohol	• Beer, drinks mixed with carbonated beverages, and red wine are particularly troublesome.
• Modify spices and seasonings	• Don't need to be eliminated. • Important for keeping food flavorful and interesting. • Use ground pepper instead of whole peppercorns, mild curry instead of hot.
• Adjust meal sizes and timing	• Eat 3 smaller meals, snacks in between. • Aim for 5–6 smaller meals per day. • Eat dinner early in the evening. Make lunch the main meal.
• Separate solids from liquids	• Consume solid food (e.g., a sandwich) and wait 30–45 minutes before consuming beverage. • Small sips of fluid with solid food is okay.
• Delay gastric emptying (provided that ileal brake mechanism is intact)	• Ileal brake is a feedback mechanism that helps to slow transit time of food through the bowel by regulating how quickly the stomach empties. • Ensure fat and protein are components of each meal. • Focus on complex carbohydrates and inclusion of soluble fiber.
• Drink oral rehydration solutions	• These fluids are superior for absorption of water across the bowel wall to help you hydrate, so include them in addition to your other fluids.

Antidiarrheal Medications

Antidiarrheal medications are another strategy that can provide some relief and help you regain some quality of life. For instance, if you are not able to sleep throughout the night due to high stool outputs, medication can be used temporarily to reduce frequency so you can sleep a little longer. Sleeping better may, in turn, help you to cope better. Examples of medications that can help to slow high stool outputs are Imodium, Lomotil, cholestyramine, and codeine phosphate.

Fluid Diets

For a short time following surgery, while experiencing obstructive symptoms, or during a flare, you may need to follow a fluid diet to relieve your symptoms by eliminating most indigestible food matter (also called residue). You might also be asked to follow a liquid-only diet if you have a fistula.

Even though you don't have much of an appetite under these conditions, you may find that you are able to drink fluids. However, while on a fluid diet, it may be difficult to consume enough calories to maintain your weight.

Clear Fluid Diets

Unfortunately, clear fluids are not a balanced source of nutrition, and are especially lacking in calories and protein. A clear fluid diet should generally be limited to no longer than several days. On this diet, you can easily develop taste fatigue and boredom with the lack of variety, texture, smell, and taste.

Examples of clear fluids are strained vegetable or meat broths, tea, coffee, clear Popsicles, Jell-O, clear juices or cocktails (such as apple or cranberry), fruit punch and other sweetened drinks, soda pop, and specially prepared nutritional products, such as Resource Fruit Beverage or Ensure Clear. Clear fluids flavored or sweetened with strained lemon juice, honey, sugar, or artificial sweeteners are considered to be fine.

Full Fluid Diets

Slightly more nutritious is the full fluid diet because of the addition of some dairy products or alternatives, such as soy milk for lactose-intolerant individuals or vegans (when all animal products are avoided). Still, it is difficult to meet protein requirements on the full fluid diet.

Examples of acceptable fluids on a full fluid diet are milk, cream, plant-based milks (soy, rice, hemp, coconut, cashew, or almond milk), plain or strained yogurt, strained hot cereals (oatmeal, cream of wheat), pudding, custard, ice cream, frozen yogurt, sorbet, gelato, strained cream soups, fruit juices, vegetable juice, and nutritional products that are "creamier" in texture (for example, Ensure, Boost, Resource, and pharmacy house brands).

Fluid Diet Challenges

The challenge with fluid diets is getting enough nutrition, because most fluids aren't balanced with adequate vitamins, minerals, protein, and other essential nutrients.

Maintaining Hydration and Electrolyte Balance

The more fluid you lose in your stool, the more likely you are to experience dehydration. If you have had your colon removed (where fluid and electrolytes are primarily absorbed), your small intestine will partially adapt to take over this function, but this takes time, and the stool will become pasty at best. When passing frequent liquid stool, be sure that you are getting adequate fluids and replacing electrolytes.

Best Fluids

Fluids that are best absorbed match the concentration, or osmolality, of your body fluids. This allows for the best absorption or transfer of fluid across the cell membranes in your intestine. Oral rehydration solutions (ORS) are good replacement fluids. Examples of these are Gastrolyte for adults or Pedialyte for children. Milk, juices, and sports drinks (such as Gatorade or Powerade) are not absorbed as well due to their higher sugar content and consequent higher osmolality (a measure of the concentration of molecules dissolved in water).

Water may be better absorbed than the sugary drinks, such as juices. When there is a high sugar concentration in a fluid, drinking it results in fluid shifting into the intestine from the tissues, instead of out of the intestine into the tissues and the bloodstream, thereby leading to more watery stool. You can try diluting concentrated sugar sources, such as juices and sports drinks, and sip them slowly to avoid the problem of increased diarrhea. There also are some reduced-sugar sports drinks available; these are sweetened with artificial sweeteners instead of sugar.

Also beware of fluids that are known to increase urine production and loss of water from the body — otherwise known as a diuretic effect. Examples of these fluids include caffeinated beverages and alcohol. Caffeinated beverages include dark colas (Coke, Pepsi, house-brand colas, and some root beer) and clear soft drinks (Mountain Dew), coffee, tea (including green tea), chocolate, and hot chocolate. Some medications, such as over-the-counter cold and flu remedies, also contain caffeine.

Electrolytes

Sodium and potassium are two electrolytes critical for regulation and balance of body fluids. They can be found in many foods in small amounts, but it is best to target higher sources on a regular basis if there is any concern with dehydration risk.

> **Dehydration Symptoms**
>
> Symptoms of dehydration and electrolyte loss include fatigue, feeling light-headed or faint, increased thirst, dry mouth, stomach cramps, and decreased urine output, to name a few. A rapid loss in weight from day to day is another indicator of dehydration.

Sodium and Potassium Sources

Mineral	Source
Sodium	• Bouillon cubes • Canned fish (e.g., tuna, salmon, sardines, anchovies) and dried fish (e.g., dried cod or herring) • Canned legumes • Canned soups and vegetables • Fast foods • Processed foods (e.g., processed cheese, processed and smoked meats) • Ready-to-eat cereals (e.g., instant oatmeal) • Sauces and condiments (e.g., soy, Worcestershire, and barbecue sauces, salad dressings, ketchup, relish, pickles) • Snack foods (e.g., pretzels, salted crackers, potato chips, salted popcorn, corn chips) • Table salt • Tomato sauce
Potassium	• Apricots • Asparagus • Avocados • Bananas • Barley • Beets • Brown sugar • Chocolate • Coconut water • Juices (orange, carrot, tomato, vegetable, passion fruit) • Legumes (chickpeas, lentils, split peas, kidney beans, soybeans) • Mangos • Maple syrup • Melons (cantaloupe, honeydew, watermelon) • Molasses • Nectarines • Okra • Oranges • Parsnips • Potatoes • Pumpkin • Salt substitute • Smooth nut butters • Strong tea and coffee • Sweet potatoes/yams • Tomato products (soup, sauce, paste)

Food Fears

If you've lived for a long time with an intestinal stricture and diet restrictions, it can be daunting to try new foods again after surgery has removed the stricture. If you have ever experienced a bowel obstruction as a result of the food you have eaten, the motivation to avoid pain and just "stay away" from suspicious or questionable foods is quite strong. It is normal to feel apprehensive about liberalizing your diet again, but slowly, with time, you will feel more comfortable with the function of your gut's new anatomy and digestion. It is important to chew food slowly and thoroughly, to eat small portion sizes, and to retry one new food at a time.

One goal of diet modifications is to facilitate an improved relationship with food and eating. All strategies that potentially restrict the types and varieties of foods should be reassessed periodically so they can be adjusted and a regular diet can be resumed.

Sometimes, despite your best efforts, diet modifications just do not have the desired effect. This could mean that your disease is active and requires medical therapy.

Nutrition Support

If there is risk of developing malnutrition or progression of malnutrition, sometimes a more intensive and defined form of nutrition, called nutrition support, is required. There are two types of nutrition support, total enteral nutrition (tube feeding) and total parenteral nutrition (intravenous feeding).

Tube Feeding

By itself, total enteral nutrition (TEN) can reduce the amount of inflammation in the intestine and thereby avoid the need for medications, such as steroids, that may have numerous undesirable side effects. It also has the added benefit of enhancing growth in children.

A relatively soft, small tube is passed through the nose and through the esophagus, ending up in the stomach or upper part of the small intestine. Tube feeding can be delivered by using gravity drip or a pump to deliver a precise volume per hour. Tube feeding does not preclude taking other fluids by mouth, so you can continue to drink even while you have the tube inserted.

TEN

In total enteral nutrition, nutritional supplements are delivered via a feeding tube when you are just not able to consume enough by mouth. This method of nutrition support is particularly helpful in children with certain forms of IBD, particularly Crohn's disease of the small intestine.

Children often learn how to place this tube themselves. They insert the tube every evening before going to bed, administer the feeds overnight while they sleep, and take the tube out in the morning before going about their usual activities during the day.

The procedure should be supervised by your health-care team to ensure that possible side effects of tube feeding (bloating, cramping, diarrhea) are monitored and properly addressed. There is also a cost associated with tube feeding, which is not always covered by governments or third parties, such as insurance companies.

Intravenous Nutrition

Total parenteral nutrition (TPN) is a specialized form of nutrition delivered via an intravenous line. A PICC (peripherally inserted central catheter) line is an example of a type of line that is commonly placed to deliver the concentrated nutrients to a large blood vessel, which rapidly dilutes the solution. In this kind of nutrition support, the gut can rest because no absorption is required while nutrients are delivered directly into the bloodstream.

TPN may be required before surgery if you are very ill and cannot consume enough nutrition by mouth or by tube feeding. Sometimes after surgery the bowel is slow to work; TPN can be provided until this resolves and you are eating well again. With multiple surgeries for Crohn's disease, some individuals don't have enough length of intestine left to absorb adequate nutrients and maintain stable weight, fluid balance, and electrolyte balance. These people may need TPN permanently, in which case there are home TPN programs available in many communities to prescribe and monitor the administration of TPN.

This may seem like a perfect solution to avoid the discomfort of gastrointestinal intolerance symptoms from eating. Besides the high cost, there are, however, risks that need to be taken into account before making a decision to use TPN. These include a higher risk of infection, blood clots (deep vein thrombosis), and metabolic intolerance. Because this is an artificial way to provide nutrition, your body often has difficulty processing the nutrients, and you could develop problems with your liver or gallbladder or abnormalities of cholesterol, triglycerides, and sugar levels in the blood as a result. Some people do not feel hungry while on TPN because the intravenous solution is giving them enough calories, but they sometimes do psychologically miss eating food and want to eat.

A specialized nutrition support team can help to avoid these complications while monitoring and adjusting the TPN to account for blood values that are unstable or abnormal.

| **TPN** |
| In total parenteral nutrition, nutrients in a solution are administered directly into a person's vein by means of an intravenous line. |

Nutrition Research

Many people are hopeful that nutrition may play a role not only in treating but also in preventing IBD. There are several areas of research that hold this promise.

Synbiotics

"Synbiotics" refers to both prebiotics and probiotics, which contribute to maintaining the health of the intestinal bacteria and keep a sufficient number of "good" bacteria in the intestine.

Bacteria in the intestinal tract is an important factor in maintaining an appropriate balance within the body's immune system. The inflammatory response is actually a natural protective mechanism, but can be damaging if it is overactive or uncontrolled. It is thought that some of the "good" bacteria normally present in the intestine contribute to maintaining the appropriate balance of the immune response.

There are food and supplement sources of both prebiotics and probiotics, but how much and how often you should eat these foods to experience benefits is not known.

Prebiotics

Prebiotics are nondigestible carbohydrates that are fermented by colonic bacteria. The process of fermentation provides energy for the growth of "good" bacteria, which, in turn, produce short-chain fatty acids, which are a fuel source for the cells lining the large intestine. Prebiotics also promote water and electrolyte reabsorption.

Prebiotics known as fructo-oligosaccharides (FOS) can be found in everyday foods, such as onions, bananas, tomatoes, honey, garlic, barley, and wheat. Some nutrition companies are adding these prebiotics to their food supplement drinks and puddings.

More recently, food companies have been adding a prebiotic named inulin (a soluble fiber processed from chicory root) to dairy products, chocolate, and beverages. Interestingly, most soluble fibers, including psyllium fiber, are considered prebiotics.

Probiotics

Probiotics are any number of different "good" live bacteria that are administered by mouth, in a capsule or in a drink or food, and confer a health benefit. The bacteria then establish themselves and grow within the intestine, a process called colonization. They are thought to provide immune system balance by downregulating inflammation.

> **Limits**
>
> As with all fermentable foods, be sure to limit your intake of prebiotics to only a few grams a day in order to avoid gas and cramping. When foods are fermented by bacteria in the intestine, gas is produced as a normal by-product. Although not abnormal, gas may be uncomfortable or difficult to manage in some social situations.

Live bacteria are most easily found in yogurts and kefir, where active bacterial cultures have been added. Unfortunately, there is no standardization regarding the bacterial strains or amount of bacterial colony forming units (CFUs) added. Similarly, the amount of remaining live bacteria when you consume the product will be affected by the processing, transport, and storage conditions. Live bacteria need to be kept in a refrigerated environment. Probiotics must also arrive alive in the gut, so they must be acid- and bile-resistant.

Examples of probiotics include *Lactobacillus acidophilus* and bifidobacterium. When buying yogurt, look for those that "contain" active cultures as compared with those that are "made with" active cultures to be sure you're getting as much of the live bacteria as possible. It is important to know the strain of bacteria because not all strains in a given group have the same benefit.

Immunonutrition (Omega-3 Fatty Acids)

This rapidly expanding area of nutrition is of interest wherever there is an inflammatory component to disease (for example, arthritis, cardiovascular disease, IBD). Immunonutrition involves modulating the inflammatory response through diet. The type of fat we eat is directly related to the fat that makes up our cells, which influences a cell's ability to produce eicosanoids and cytokines. These are hormonelike compounds that affect the body's immune response to injury and infection. By eating more anti-inflammatory fats, we can directly influence production of these anti-inflammatory mediators.

There are a few different kinds of dietary fats, including trans fats, saturated fats, monounsaturated fats, and polyunsaturated fats (PUFAs), including the essential omega-3 and omega-6 PUFAs. "Essential" means that our body cannot make those fatty acids and we can get them only through our diet. Two important omega-3 fatty acids are eicosapentaenoic acid (EPA) and docosahexaenoic acid (DHA). You will get these from fish and seafood. Another omega-3 fatty acid is alpha-linolenic acid (ALA), and you get this from plant-based foods.

Optimal Dose

The optimal amount of omega-3 in the diet has not been defined in IBD. In cardiovascular disease, the optimal intake has been defined as 1000 mg EPA plus DHA per day. For the general public, some recommendations in the medical literature suggest an intake of 400 to 500 mg per day as being optimal. While ALA is not as efficiently converted to EPA and DHA in the body, it is still recommended (National Academy of Sciences) that women need 1100 mg, and men 1600 mg per day.

Anti-Inflammatory Fats

Omega-3 fats are anti-inflammatory, while omega-6 are pro-inflammatory. In North America, our balance between these two essential fats is skewed, and we generally consume too much omega-6 and not enough omega-3 fats.

To put this in perspective, one omega-3 egg has roughly 5 mg EPA and 75 mg DHA. Omega-3 milk has roughly 15 mg DHA per cup (250 mL). Some of these products have added costs, so be sure to read the label to determine whether the additional omega-3 is significant enough to add to your daily totals.

Marine sources of omega-3 are the best sources of EPA and DHA, the forms most easily used by the body. ALA from plant sources is only partially converted by the body to EPA and DHA. Still, it is considered worthwhile to include plant sources of omega-3 along with marine sources because this can improve the balance of omega-3 to omega-6 fatty acids in the diet. It is also thought that ALA may help the body's metabolism of blood sugar.

Essential Fatty Acids (Omega-6 and Omega-3) Sources

Omega-6	Omega-3
Vegetable oils • Corn oil • Cottonseed oil • Sunflower oil • Safflower oil (Can also be found in processed foods and commercial baked goods)	**Oils** • Canola oil • Chia seeds (salba seeds) • Cold water fatty fish: salmon, tuna, trout, mackerel, anchovy, sardines, sturgeon, bluefish, mullet, herring (menhaden) • Dark green leafy vegetables • Fish oil • Flaxseed oil • Functional foods: omega-3 eggs, DHA milk, soy beverages, cheese, yogurt, margarine, organic grain cereals (some of these foods contain only marginally higher amounts) • Ground flaxseed (add in baked goods, add to moist foods like yogurt, applesauce, sauces) • Hemp seeds • Krill oil • Soybeans • Walnut oil

Notes: Fish oil supplements are often made from fish skin and liver and may contain environmental contaminants. Check ingredient labels for more information. Consider omega-3 (DHA) supplements made from algae instead.

Functional foods are conventional foods (fish, for example) or those similar in appearance to a conventional food (omega-3 eggs, for example) that are part of a usual diet and that demonstrate a physiological health benefit.

CASE STUDY James

James is a 34-year-old man who has been living with ulcerative colitis for 7 years. Although his symptoms initially responded to 5-ASA therapy, over the years, the flares no longer responded as well and he required several courses of prednisone. Eventually, he was placed on an immunosuppressant drug, azathioprine, to try to keep his colitis in remission and avoid the need for more courses of prednisone. Overall, azathioprine seemed to reduce how frequently he experienced flares but did not completely eliminate them.

James was not entirely satisfied with the results of his medical treatment and wanted to consider other options, such as diet, for controlling his condition. He booked an appointment with his gastroenterologist, who told him there was no role for diet in treating ulcerative colitis and said he should simply stick with the prescribed medication. She also suggested that, if James wasn't happy with how he was doing, he could consider going on one of the biologic drugs.

He left the doctor's office feeling frustrated. His partner had recently decided to try a new diet for its general health benefits. The diet was supposed to have anti-inflammatory properties, so James figured it might help his colitis, since colitis is an inflammatory disease. With his partner following the diet too, James found that sticking to it wasn't as difficult as he'd thought it might be. After a week or two on the diet, he was feeling a bit better, although his bowel function had not really changed. At that point, he decided to stop taking azathioprine.

James continued on the diet and has felt well for about 9 months. Over that time, he has lost about 11 pounds (5 kg), even though he would not have been considered overweight beforehand. Recently, he has started to have some diarrhea, blood in his stool, and abdominal cramping. He worries that he is experiencing a colitis flare and has started asking himself a number of questions: Is this really a flare of his colitis? If it is, is it happening because he is not following his diet properly? Are there foods he is eating that he shouldn't be, or are there foods he should be eating more of? Could this be happening because he stopped taking azathioprine? Should he go back to see his doctor, or will she be angry that he decided to go on the diet and stop his medication?

James does return to his doctor, and she reinforces the concept that diet alone cannot be relied on to prevent flares of colitis. She suggests that the diet might have worked better if it was used in combination with other forms of therapy, such as the medication he stopped taking. She also points out that James's unintended weight loss might reflect an imbalance in the diet. She advises him to consult with a registered dietitian if he wishes to pursue further diet therapy, to ensure that he is eating the right amount and proportion of various nutrients. She also stresses that the colitis flare is not his fault and was not caused by a failure to stick with his diet, reminding him that flares often occur without apparent cause.

Antioxidants

The area of antioxidants and IBD looks promising, but studies are still at a biochemical level and cannot yet be translated to specific recommendations for people. Antioxidants include vitamin E, vitamin C, carotenoids, glutathione, and selenium.

An Anti-Inflammatory Diet

Antioxidants and fish oils may have beneficial effects on the immune system and inflammation. There may also be other foods, or components of foods, that help to maintain appropriate immune response and reduce inflammation. Attempts have been made to tie this theory into an overall dietary program recommendation — called an anti-inflammatory diet — rather than a single dietary supplement. The diet contains foods such as fish (particularly those higher in omega-3), fruits (primarily blueberries, blackberries, strawberries, and raspberries), vegetables, beans, nuts and seeds, and olive oil. The diet also avoids or limits processed foods. There is research being carried out to determine if following this type of diet will reduce inflammation in people living with IBD, but as yet there is no conclusive answer.

Diet Counseling

While there is no standard diet for IBD, diet modifications can help with symptom management. Diet restrictions are usually temporary during times of disease activity or postoperative recovery periods.

Any diet modifications should be discussed with your doctor or dietitian. Changes to usual food choices need to be practical and realistic, while taking into consideration individual choices for reasons of religion, culture, ethnicity, beliefs, personal food preferences, tolerances, allergies, phobias, lifestyle, employment, sports, and financial considerations. This is why diet modifications aren't just about changing something like fiber in your diet; they are individualized recommendations that work for you as an individual living with IBD.

CHAPTER 6

Psychological Support for Managing IBD

Dr. Bob Maunder and Dr. A. Hillary Steinhart

CASE STUDIES Susan and Jerome

Susan is 22, in her fourth year of university. She was diagnosed with ulcerative colitis at the age of 17. She is frustrated with the course of her disease. Diarrhea, fatigue, and the medication she takes all seem to interfere with her concentration at school. She has decided that she wants to look into pelvic pouch surgery, but doesn't know whether she should take more time off school for the operation or try to schedule it in the summer break. "I never know whether I am pushing myself too hard," she tells her doctor, "or if I just need to keep trying to live a normal life at a normal pace."

Jerome, 42, teaches at a high school and has been living with Crohn's disease for 20 years. Given the time constraints of his job, he used to find it difficult to get through the day without interruption or fear of embarrassment. In recent years, he has found strategies to cope with these pressures. "I don't have any choice about what time I start my day," he explains. "Mornings are usually tricky for me because I'm likely to have to go to the bathroom a few times before 9:00. It used to be more of a stress, but now I eat a smaller breakfast and drive to work instead of taking the bus, so I'm less likely to have to go really badly, and if I do, I can stop at a public washroom. I know where all of the washrooms are on my route to work!"

Psychological Concerns

Once considered by some health-care professionals as psychosomatic illnesses, we now know that Crohn's disease and ulcerative colitis are not caused by personality or other psychological factors. Although we have learned a great deal about the experience of living with inflammatory bowel disease, there is much that we don't yet understand about the relationship between mind and body. One thing is certain: if you have inflammatory bowel disease, you should pay attention to what is happening to you emotionally during the course of your illness and how the illness affects your life and your relationships.

The range of psychological issues relevant to IBD is large. Some challenges affect almost everybody with IBD to some extent. These include finding ways to live with the uncertainty inherent in the disease. Other common challenges are tolerating physical symptoms, such as fatigue and pain, and dealing with the ways the disease affects relationships, ranging from concerns about the way that embarrassment may affect day-to-day relationships to concerns about burdening friends and family at times when you need to depend on them. Some challenges may not affect all people with IBD but require extra attention, such as the role of stress in triggering a flare of inflammation, or complications leading to depression.

Developing strategies for relieving and preventing stress and depression is important for managing IBD and improving your quality of life. The fundamental strategy is to know yourself. Think about your experience with health problems and with other challenges in your life. What have you done that has helped in the past? What has been less successful? Who in your life has been most supportive? Where can you turn for support? We'll help you answer these questions.

Quality of Life

While psychological factors do not cause your disease and while psychological changes will not cure it, your mental attitude and the way that you understand your illness can contribute significantly to your quality of life. Seek psychological support from health-care professionals, family members, and friends to manage your condition.

Psychological Factors in IBD Management

Besides coping with the pain and fatigue your disease may be causing, there are other psychological factors that may cause considerable discomfort. In more serious cases, these factors may lead to chronic stress, anxiety, and depression.

Uncertainty: How can I predict the course of my disease hour to hour, day to day, and month to month? When will the next flare occur?

Embarrassment: How do I talk about this disease with family, friends, and acquaintances when bowel symptoms are not usually part of polite conversation?

Anxiety: How do I find or keep a romantic partner when I have a bowel disease?

Worry: What physical and mental abilities will be affected by the disease? Will I be able to maintain my family, social, work, and educational responsibilities?

Adjustment: What adjustments will I need to make to my plans for the future?

Dependence: Are my loved ones going to get tired of me if I depend on them too much?

Guilt: Am I trying hard enough? Did something I do cause this disease or this flare?

Doubt: Is it okay to ask for help?

Q **What is the role of stress in IBD?**

A Scientific research into the role of stress in triggering flares of illness in patients with Crohn's disease or ulcerative colitis is about evenly split between studies that find a link and studies that find no link between stress and these diseases. These studies have shown the following evidence, however:

- Personality has no impact on whether or not a person develops IBD.
- Life stresses probably have no impact on whether or not a person develops IBD.
- Life stress may be one of the factors that can trigger a flare of disease when disease has been inactive, but this is probably only true for some people with IBD.

Stress

While stress does not cause Crohn's disease or ulcerative colitis, these conditions do cause stress for patients and their families. Coping with pain, fatigue, and potentially embarrassing symptoms, as well as complicated decisions about treatment, clearly can be stressful, but some of the strongest sources of stress for people with IBD are less obvious.

Patient perception of the role of stress is also split. About 1 in 3 people with IBD believes that stress or psychological factors had something to do with getting the illness in the first place. About 3 in 4 people believe that stress affects the course of their disease.

In determining whether stress is a factor in your IBD, try to distinguish between experiencing common gut symptoms and active inflammation (a flare of disease). An increase in symptoms does not always mean that the intestine is inflamed. You can experience increased fatigue, pain, or diarrhea for many reasons other than IBD. In fact, these symptoms of an irritable bowel are quite common in IBD even when there is no active inflammation. There is some evidence that once a person's bowel has been affected by repeated occurrences of inflammation and healing, it is more likely to respond to stress with diarrhea and pain, even if a flare of inflammation doesn't occur.

Until there is better evidence upon which to base decisions, the best policy seems to be to know yourself and trust your experience. If you believe from your own experience with IBD that the stresses in your life (or the way that you react to them) have an impact on your symptoms, then it makes sense to try to modify the ways that you respond to stress. If your experience is that your disease course doesn't seem to depend on what is happening in your life, then you are probably right.

Maintaining Your Resilience to Stress

- Try to maintain a stable, predictable pattern of sleep, healthy diet, and moderate exercise. Although the symptoms of IBD may make it challenging to eat, exercise, and sleep, these can be powerful tools to maximize your health. It is very hard to manage stress effectively when you are sleep-deprived or malnourished.
- Try to identify and fix problems as they occur. The trick to this strategy is that it is usually the constructive effort to try to solve a problem that reduces stress, rather than the solution itself. Don't focus single-mindedly on the outcome of your efforts.
- Try to accept and tolerate the problems that can't be fixed. Whether or not you are religious, remember the Serenity Prayer: **God, grant me the serenity to accept the things I cannot change, the courage to change the things I can, and the wisdom to know the difference.**
- Keep a sense of humor.
- Engage with life. Be an active part of your family, your circle of friends, and your community.
- Attend to your spiritual needs.
- Learn and use relaxation techniques or meditation.
- Take time for leisure.
- Avoid caffeine.

Depression

Depression is a very common illness. It would be surprising if you did not know someone who has lived with depression, since approximately 1 in 5 women and 1 in 10 men will experience a major depression at some point in their life. Depression is different from normal sadness or discouragement because it has a wider range of effects on feeling, thinking, and physical function, and because, if not treated, it usually persists for weeks or months.

People who live with chronic diseases, such as IBD, are at increased risk of experiencing depression. There are probably many reasons for the increased risk. The losses and frustrations that come with living with a disease; the biological effects of inflammation (since many of the body's chemicals that increase immunity and inflammation also have effects on the brain); and the effects of medications, such as prednisone, may all contribute to depression.

Successful Treatments

Fortunately, depression can be treated effectively. The most effective forms of treatment are antidepressant medications, certain modes of psychotherapy or counseling, or a combination of these. If you think you are depressed, you should talk to your doctor.

Recognizing the symptoms of depression (see sidebar, page 139) when they occur is very important, because depression usually responds well to treatment. Some of these symptoms may be hard to interpret when you have ulcerative colitis or Crohn's disease. Most people experience one or two of these symptoms some of the time without being depressed. Some can be caused by physical illness without being depressed. However, if symptoms persist and seem out of proportion to your usual experience of illness, talk to your doctor about the possibility of depression. It is important to bring up your feelings and concerns because doctors often do not ask about the symptoms of depression or may consider them to be part of a patient's IBD symptoms. In some IBD clinics or doctors' practices, screening for depression using symptom questionnaires has become more routine and has allowed for more in-depth assessment and management of depression.

IBD and Depression Cycle

Changes in ability to function at work and school
Impact on family and relationships
Impact on self-image
Difficulty initiating new relationships
Loss of sense of well-being
Changes in potential for future
Sense of stigma and isolation
Biological effects of inflammation
Biological effects of IBD treatments

IBD

Depression

Difficulty remembering and taking medication
Difficulty attending medical appointments and following through with tests
Increased pain and other symptoms
Effects of treatments for depression
Reduced support from others or reduced ability to take advantage of support

Vicious Cycle

If it is not treated, depression adds substantially to the burden of illness. People with chronic disease who are also depressed tend to experience more pain, fatigue, and other symptoms. Depression makes it harder to keep up your motivation to see the doctor when IBD symptoms emerge and to stick to your treatment plan. If you are depressed, you are less likely to be able to work and you are less likely to be effective in all of your efforts to cope with IBD. The result is that depression and IBD can make each other worse in a vicious cycle.

Treating Depression

Depression can be effectively treated with antidepressant drugs or with certain forms of psychotherapy. Very often these forms of treatment are most effective if used together.

Drug Therapy

There are many effective antidepressant drugs available now. Your doctor can help you to choose the drug that is best suited to your situation.

Treating depression requires daily use of antidepressants for several months, often longer. However, depressive symptoms usually start to improve after taking an antidepressant for about 2 weeks, although it may take up to 12 weeks to feel the full benefit.

With modern antidepressant drugs, side effects (such as tremor, difficulty sleeping, or upset stomach) are usually not difficult to tolerate. Side effects are usually strongest shortly after starting a new medication or increasing the dose, and tend to settle down after a couple of weeks. Your doctor can help you to find a drug that is compatible with your IBD symptoms and its treatment.

Psychotherapy

Some forms of psychotherapy (talk therapy) are as effective as antidepressant drugs for treating moderately severe depression. Cognitive-behavioral therapy and interpersonal therapy, for example, have been found to be highly effective in many studies of depression. Other forms of psychotherapy may also be effective.

In cognitive-behavioral therapy, you learn to identify patterns of thought that tend to lead to depression or that tend to make depressive feelings worse. It is very common for people with depression to evaluate their experience in a

> **Common Symptoms of Depression**
>
> - Lack of interest in things that are usually interesting to you
> - Feeling excessively guilty or sad
> - "Low" mood that doesn't improve when circumstances improve
> - Feeling helpless about the present or hopeless about the future
> - Low self-esteem or feelings of worthlessness
> - Not participating in social activities even though you are physically well enough
> - Thinking about suicide or being preoccupied with death
> - Reduced appetite
> - Reduced energy
> - Poor concentration and memory
> - Sleep disturbance

Preparing for Psychotherapy

- Choose a therapist who makes you feel safe, comfortable, and at ease when discussing your health. You need to have a good working relationship with your therapist.

- Choose a therapist with appropriate credentials, training, and professional ethics (such as a physician, psychologist, or social worker). Ask your family doctor or a local health clinic for references.

- Keep an open mind about using psychotherapy and an antidepressant drug at the same time. A combination of psychotherapy and drug therapy has proven to be effective in treating depression.

way that leads to negative conclusions. Seeing things as black or white (all good or all bad), for example, means that many experiences and events are labeled as being bad, just because they aren't perfect. Many depressed people find that they pay close attention to negative or unhappy events and do not pay the same degree of attention to positive events, which tends to reinforce a pessimistic view. Patients work with their therapist to recognize their typical patterns of thought, to reevaluate how accurate they are, and to develop alternative modes of thought. Typically, cognitive-behavioral therapy occurs weekly for 3 or 4 months, sometimes longer.

In interpersonal therapy, patients work through, with their therapist, the feelings that are associated with an important life event linked to the current period of depression. Typical examples are grief over the death of a loved one, dealing with the mixed feelings of making a critical developmental transition (such as moving from living with family to living on your own), dealing with conflict in a partner relationship, or coping with social isolation. Interpersonal therapy also typically occurs weekly for 3 to 4 months, sometimes longer.

Coping Strengths

People differ in their coping strengths, but, in general, the ways of coping that seem to be the most productive for most people are problem-solving, seeking emotional and practical support from others, looking for the positives in challenging situations, maintaining realistic expectations, and keeping a sense of humor. Less successful ways of coping, in general, include pretending that there isn't a problem (denial), avoiding any response, and acting out of anger.

Coping Strategies

Much of what occurs in the course of living with IBD is not precisely under your control. Try to focus your attention on the things that you can control and use these to your advantage. Your own individual style of relating to yourself and to others may have a big influence on how you experience disease. So it is helpful to know your behavioral style and how it may affect your experience of IBD.

Relationship Questionnaire
(adapted from Dr. Kim Bartholomew)

Look at these four basic interpersonal styles and see which one is the closest match to your style. Check the description that is closest to your relationship style.

Adaptable
It's easy for me to become emotionally close to others. I'm comfortable depending on them and having them depend on me. I don't worry about being alone or having others not accept me.

Support-seeking
I want to be completely emotionally intimate with others, but I often find that others are reluctant to get as close as I would like. I'm uncomfortable being without close relationships, but I sometimes worry that others don't value me as much as I value them.

Self-reliant
I'm comfortable without close emotional relationships. It's very important to me to feel independent and self-sufficient, and I prefer not to depend on others or have others depend on me.

Cautious
I'm uncomfortable getting close to others. I want emotionally close relationships, but I find it difficult to trust others completely or to depend on them. I worry that I will be hurt if I allow myself to become too close to others.

1. Know Your Interpersonal Style

One useful way of describing personal style is to look at how you prefer to relate to the people who are closest to you at times of stress. Do you look for the company of your partner or family members to talk things through and to feel supported? Do you depend on others to care for you when you are feeling overwhelmed? Do you find that you want to retreat from others and handle things alone?

People differ in the way they use close relationships to feel comfortable and secure at times of stress, and these differences have an impact on medical care. The impact of interpersonal style on medical care has received careful study in the last few years. Bear in mind that many things in addition to interpersonal style determine health outcomes.

Easy to Work With

Depending on how you measure things, about 30% to 60% of people have an adaptable interpersonal style. Health-care professionals usually report that it is easy to work with someone with an adaptable style, even if the medical situation is complicated.

Adaptable Style

The adaptable style is usually associated with relative ease in using medical resources because people with this style tend to be comfortable with independence and with depending on others. Adaptable individuals are usually comfortable monitoring their situation independently and making their own health choices. They are also able to turn to others for assistance when the situation demands.

Support-Seeking Style

People with the support-seeking style are more comfortable and may function more effectively when the people they count upon for support are near. People with a support-seeking style who have very supportive people in their life look and act very similar to people with an adaptable style. However, without good support from others, a person with a support-seeking style may be troubled by worry and negative feelings.

In general, the support-seeking style is associated with reporting more intense symptoms and a greater number of symptoms (including ones that aren't typical for IBD or due to IBD). The support-seeking style is associated with more frequent visits to the doctor, and more tests. This may relate to a greater need for reassurance from others in order to feel comfortable. When IBD is active, the support-seeking style is associated with a higher risk of depression. Doctors of support-seeking patients find it easier to appreciate the significance of the changes in the course of IBD when they have known each other long enough for the doctor to recognize the patient's style of communication. Otherwise, there is a risk of overestimating the current level or severity of disease activity.

Self-Reliant Style

The self-reliant style is characterized by the lowest levels of symptom reporting. Visits to the doctor are infrequent. When it comes to one's health, a self-reliant interpersonal style may be a positive or a negative influence.

When managing diseases that require a great deal of collaboration between patients and health-care professionals, a self-reliant style can interfere, especially when patients do not disclose the whole picture of their current state or when a lack of collaboration is frustrating for the patient or the health-care provider. Doctors may need to schedule regular visits or tests rather than wait for a self-reliant patient to decide it is time to check in.

Self-Reliance Benefits and Risks

There is some evidence that self-reliant individuals have better health outcomes for some conditions. However, self-reliant individuals are prone to follow their own advice rather than seeking a professional opinion and may suffer silently with symptoms for longer than is reasonable.

Cautious Style

The cautious style includes a push and pull when it comes to dealing with others, which can be tricky to balance in a medical setting. When a level of discomfort in managing things on one's own is combined with cautiousness about being willing to approach others or depend on them for help, a person with the cautious style may sometimes feel stuck.

These people are similar to self-reliant people in their relative underutilization of medical resources (preferring, for example, not to go to the doctor if it can be avoided), but are like people with a support-seeking style in their relatively greater experience of symptoms. If the situation calls for trying to overcome cautiousness, many people find it easiest to do this by finding one or two close confidants and relying on them to help with the challenges involved in being ill.

Depression Risk
Like the support-seeking style, when IBD is active, people with a cautious style are at greater risk of becoming depressed.

2. Know Your Information-Gathering Style

A second way of understanding your behavioral style is to pay attention to how much information you like to have about your health. There is no right or wrong approach, but there are two main styles of collecting information, known to some psychologists as monitors or blunters. It helps to know your information-gathering style because most of the time you will be most comfortable if you stick to your own style. It is also helpful to be aware of the ways in which these styles may lead to trouble if you overdo it.

Monitors

Some people feel most comfortable when they know everything. They prefer to monitor small changes in how they are feeling. They like to get opinions about what may be going on and what all the options are to treat their illness. Monitors often spend time on the Internet keeping up on the latest developments and researching all aspects of their medications. Monitors often find that it is comforting to gather more information (even if they don't end up acting on it).

Information-Gathering Risks
The risk for monitors is that they will continue to gather information when it is no longer serving any useful purpose. For example, after you have gathered all of the information you need to make informed decisions, further exhaustive Internet searches of dubious sources of information can raise anxiety rather than awareness. The risk for blunters is that they may not gather enough information to be well-informed about their choices.

Taking Control of your IBD

Problem-Solving Strategies
- Get information
- Weigh your options
- Choose your best course
- Reevaluate

Helpful Attitudes
- Look for the positives in challenging situations
- Maintain realistic expectations
- Keep a sense of humor

Many of these general rules depend on context, of course. The difference between having a sense of humor about events that aren't very funny and denying the reality of your situation is only a matter of degree. Similarly, the difference between the healthy assertiveness of insisting on your rights as a health consumer versus angry hostility toward those who want to help is a difference that may be in the eye of the beholder.

Blunters

Other people want information only on a need-to-know basis. Blunters are often content to let their health-care providers recommend choices and don't want to know all of the details behind each choice. They may find that gathering extra information is anxiety-provoking rather than comforting. "Why should I hear about all of the things that might happen in the future? I'd rather just deal with things as they come up" is something that a blunter might say.

3. Know When Stress Is Beyond Your Comfort Zone

Often people respond to challenges that feel within their grasp through problem-solving and persistence, but respond to circumstances that are beyond their personal resources with emotional distress — feelings of grief, panic, or giving up. These are normal responses to extraordinary circumstances and shouldn't be interpreted as a sign of personal weakness or failure.

When stress feels like it is passing beyond your comfort zone, it is time to step back and reassess your options. Review the situation to see if the problem-solving strategies and helpful attitudes that usually work for you might work in this situation as well. Consider new ways of coping. For example, if you are a person who usually perseveres through trouble with a stiff upper lip, maybe now is a time to consider allowing yourself a breather and asking for help. In general, when stress crosses beyond the limits of your comfort zone, it is a good idea to consider allowing others to help.

Scripts for Improving Communication

- Others may offer to help but not know what to do. If someone says that they would like to help, offer something practical to do that is helpful to you.

  Thank you. Can you watch my kids next Thursday morning so that I can go to this appointment?

- Speak for yourself. Avoid blame. Describe the feeling and the event, not the person.

  I feel uncomfortable seeing the surgeon by myself. Can you come with me? This may be more effective than saying *Why haven't you offered to come to the surgeon with me?* And it's much more effective than going to the surgeon alone without asking.

4. Turn to Others

Often, at times of crisis, it is very helpful to call upon the support of others, including family and friends who can offer practical support and can "be there for you" emotionally as good listeners. Moral support and practical help are usually more valuable than free advice. Professionals may be able to offer treatment and management options that have not been considered, which may also help to move illness challenges back into the realm where they feel manageable again.

Recognizing Obstacles

You have many resources to draw upon to help you with the challenges of illness, including your family and friends, health-care professionals, peer support groups, and your community. Sometimes you may want to turn to others, but you experience obstacles. Pay attention to these obstacles to see what is within your control. If you feel that you cannot turn to others for support, ask yourself why. Why are you reluctant to depend on someone else? Do you feel guilty burdening them? Were you disappointed in how they responded in the past? Many people face challenges of this kind, especially with partners, close friends, and family. You probably need to identify the type of obstacle you are experiencing before you can overcome it.

Opportunities for Kindness

Telling others about your disease can be a liberating, rather than an embarrassing, experience. Many people are sympathetic to your condition and respond to your confidence in them with acts of extraordinary kindness, as Robert Mason Lee, a celebrated author with Crohn's disease, observes:

"People are always telling me that because I have Crohn's disease I shouldn't be doing the fun things they are doing — like having a beer, for example, or eating something other than brown rice. It is hugely annoying, because almost without exception these people do not know what they are talking about, recommending foods I know would leave me in hospital or warning me away from foods that I enjoy. I do my best to forgive these people for their helpful instinct, because I understand the desire to heal…

"What I have found, instead, is that just about everyone is good at offering comfort. I have had the hands of compassion laid upon me by doctors, nurses, ambulance attendants, the women in my life, friends, the wives of friends, complete strangers in bus terminals. When it comes to offering solace, people have a natural ability which transcends social place or relationships. We just give, naturally, of ourselves to those in need.

"One small consolation of having such a painful illness is the many opportunities it allows others to show kindness; the one great reassurance is how seldom I have been disappointed."

Improving Communication

Clear communication is often your most powerful tool. It helps you to sort the real differences in opinion and conflicts that you experience with others from the ones that are based on your assumptions and expectations. Clear communication may also help to change a conflict that feels irremediable ("You always avoid me when I am in pain. I think you are insensitive…") to a problem that can be negotiated ("I want to help you, but I don't know how. When you are in pain, you stop talking and I feel powerless to help…").

Managing Medical Meetings and Appointments

Many people find medical visits to be stressful, especially when things are changing — when there are new symptoms or a new diagnosis, or a new treatment is being considered. Anxiety and stress make it harder to pay attention and take in all of the information that is being discussed. The stress of the situation also makes it harder to retain the composure that you need to ask your questions and make sure that they are answered.

Try to anticipate what you want to get out of a meeting with your doctor or specialist and prepare yourself accordingly.

- Make sure there is enough time. Make an appointment to address your concerns instead of trying to find a moment at the end of another conversation.
- Make a list of your questions. Keep it short enough that it can realistically be covered in the available time.
- Bring a friend or relative to help you remember what you have discussed.
- Take notes.

Community Support

Crohn's and Colitis Foundations

There are several organizations in North America that, in addition to raising money for research, also provide education and support to patients and families. Two such organizations are the Crohn's and Colitis Foundation (CCF) in the United States and Crohn's and Colitis Canada (CCC). Although the national offices of these organizations may not provide individuals with the type of small group support and personal contact that they are looking for, the local chapters are often a good way to network with other patients and families dealing with IBD.

Internet Resources

The availability of other community support varies from location to location, but many patients and families turn to the Internet, where there are numerous means of communication with other individuals who are in situations similar to your own. However, you should be careful about the quality of the information and support that you might find in places like Internet chat rooms or blogs. Typically, chat rooms are not monitored by someone with the necessary expertise who can put the information and opinions provided into proper perspective or context. If you hear or read something unusual, something disturbing, or something that just doesn't seem right, you should discuss it with your doctor.

In addition, remember that, although IBD is considered a single group of diseases, its presentation and response to treatment can be completely different from one person to the next. As a result, what one person experienced or a treatment that helped someone may not necessarily apply to you. These Internet sites do provide an opportunity for you to discuss your thoughts, feelings, and hopes with others, particularly if you find it difficult to do so face-to-face. The responses that you get may not always make you feel better, but, in many cases, people are able to find some comfort in describing their situation and knowing that there are others in similar situations.

Coping with the Medical System

Navigating through the medical system successfully can be a stressful challenge in itself. Having a chronic disease means that over time you will likely need to make use of a variety of medical resources, including hospitals, clinics, and laboratories. You are also likely to come in contact with a wide range of professionals in these settings — nurses, dietitians, enterostomal therapy nurses, family doctors, gastroenterologists, surgeons, emergency department staff, pharmacists, and many others are often helpful along the way. Some will be seasoned experts and some will be students full of enthusiasm and recent knowledge.

Communication and Coping Strategies

Treating pain and other symptoms appropriately is a common challenge for many people with IBD and may easily become a source of conflict and miscommunication with health-care professionals. Most medical care starts with a conversation in which patients try to explain their symptoms, while the doctor tries to listen, understand, and explain the available options. Then patient and doctor try to come to an agreement about how to proceed. Such a conversation amounts to a negotiation — and negotiations are difficult in a context of pain and stress. A conversation about the use of pain medication that does not also treat the underlying IBD that is causing the pain can be particularly difficult because of the potential serious side effects of many pain medications and the risk of dependency or addiction. This is discussed in more detail in the next chapter.

Fortunately, when both parties negotiate in good faith, which is almost always the case, it is not hard to build an alliance and face the problem as a team.

Strategies for coping are also needed when you're undergoing drug and surgical treatments. Use your strengths to face these challenges. Others around you — friends, acquaintances, family members, or health-care professionals — will often be helpful if you are able to tell them what is wrong and how they can best help you.

> ### Treatment Challenges
>
> At times, getting the most comfortable and effective treatment for your IBD will challenge your ability to be an effective advocate for your own rights and interests, to work collaboratively with others (including times when there is disagreement), and to make the best use of the resources and supports that are available to you.

A Visit to the ER

To illustrate the complex forces that are at work between a patient and a doctor, imagine what looks on the surface to be a fairly straightforward case: Jane, who has Crohn's disease, goes to the emergency department because of intense abdominal pain. She wants to know what is going on and she needs relief. She is seen by Dr. Smith. This looks like a relatively uncomplicated medical situation, surely one that occurs quite often, but other factors make it a frustrating and difficult experience. Consider the following possibilities:

- Abdominal pain has been a chronic part of Jane's experience for years now. Although chronic pain hurts just as much as acute (sudden) pain, it doesn't look the same. People with chronic pain are not as likely to be pale and sweating, pacing or writhing, rocking in their seats, or making the noises that people with acute pain tend to make. The consequence is that Jane's pain may not look as severe as it feels.

- Jane has no way of knowing how the intensity of her pain compares to what other people experience. It is the nature of "invisible" symptoms that we have no objective yardstick to measure them. Many people are unsure of when to ask for help and when to tough it out. Unfortunately, these choices are heavy with value judgments. No one wants to be considered a wimp or a bother. But neither should anyone accept needless suffering. Jane may not be clear in her own mind that she deserves pain relief.

- Dr. Smith is well aware that there are a number of painful intestinal conditions that should not be treated with strong narcotic (opioid) pain medications, either because the drug masks the pain while the condition is getting worse (as can happen with undiagnosed appendicitis, for example, making it difficult for the health-care professionals to monitor the situation), or because the side effects of the drug can make the problem worse (as when pain medications prevent the bowel from functioning normally and aggravate an obstructed bowel).

- Dr. Smith is also aware that irritable bowel symptoms sometimes occur in the course of Crohn's disease, and so the flare of pain may or may not indicate that something has changed in Jane's gut (such as an increase in inflammation or an obstruction to the passage of the contents of the gut). Pain of that sort is called functional pain. He chooses his words carefully, because sometimes when he talks about the possibility of functional pain, his patients assume that he is telling them that the pain is "in the head."

- Dr. Smith has never met Jane before and has no way to judge her usual pain tolerance or how trustworthy or reliable she is in reporting her degree of pain. Trust and reliability are important issues because the strongest pain medications are opioids, which can be abused and cause addiction. Jane has used opioids only once before, when she was recovering from surgery. She used them as prescribed and had no difficulty stopping them after a few days when they were no longer required. Dr. Smith doesn't know this.

- Jane has never met Dr. Smith before and does not know that he is quite familiar with Crohn's disease and the treatment that she needs. She was seen by a doctor at another emergency department previously, who was dismissive and didn't seem to appreciate her condition. Her expectations of this visit are shaped by that experience to some degree, and she is aware that she is more guarded and irritable than usual when answering Dr. Smith's first few questions. It feels like she is off to a poor start, which increases her tension.

- Dr. Smith is trying to balance a number of concerns. In addition to trying to provide the best care to Jane (and the other patients in the emergency department under his care), he has a professional and legal obligation to prescribe opioid medications responsibly. Unfortunately, it is a common experience in the emergency department for persons with addictions to exaggerate complaints in order to obtain opioids. Dr. Smith's expectations of this encounter are also shaped by previous experiences.

Neither Jane nor Dr. Smith is actually thinking about **all** of the considerations in this list. But they may all be at play.

How do Jane and Dr. Smith navigate through these tricky waters? Fortunately, if this encounter goes the way of most visits to the emergency department, they will be able to communicate effectively and Jane will get the help she needs quickly. Jane will be honest and open in discussing her concerns, her current situation, and her past experiences. Dr. Smith will listen carefully and be forthright about his reasons for choosing the investigations and treatments that he believes are indicated. As with most negotiations, mutual trust and respect are the bedrock of emergency room communication, and for both parties, the best way to receive them is to give them.

It may help Jane to bring a trusted support person with her to the emergency room, who can quietly support her efforts and act on her behalf if her pain interferes with her ability to speak or care for herself. A supportive person can also act as a "backup memory" when medical information is provided, because patients in distress often find it hard to remember new information. Also, just having a friendly third party in the room often helps to prevent Jane or Dr. Smith from falling into a trap of false expectations or assumptions that complicate their exchange.

CHAPTER 7

Drug Therapy for Managing IBD

CASE STUDY Jonathan

Jonathan, the police officer with suspected Crohn's disease, underwent a number of blood and stool tests, CT enterography, and a colonoscopy. These investigations confirmed the presence of Crohn's disease involving the last part of the small intestine (ileum) and a small section of the large intestine (sigmoid colon). His doctor recommended drug therapy.

Jonathan was initially placed on budesonide and a combination of antibiotics (metronidazole and ciprofloxacin), but quickly developed a metallic taste in his mouth and persistent nausea. His gastroenterologist told him that this was probably occurring because of the metronidazole, and he advised him to cut the dose in half.

With this, Jonathan was able to continue the prescribed treatment, but though his symptoms improved somewhat, he was still experiencing episodes of mild pain and diarrhea at least 2 days out of every week and had not regained the weight he had lost.

Although the symptoms were not very bad and weren't really interfering with his work or his leisure-time activities, even biking, he wondered whether he might do better with an alternative type of therapy.

He raised this question with his doctor, and they went through the available treatment options, ranging from steroids through immunosuppressive drugs to the biologic drugs, some of which had only recently arrived on the scene. Jonathan had many questions about the likelihood of those medications providing him with additional benefit and their ability to change his long-term prognosis. He had already had the bad experience of a side effect from his relatively brief exposure to medication and was also concerned about the side effects and long-term safety of medications. Since he was feeling reasonably well at the time, he decided, after a full discussion of the available options, not to embark on any new treatment.

Treatment Goals

Before we consider the various types of drug treatments that are available for Crohn's disease and ulcerative colitis, we should have a good idea about what we are trying to achieve when we embark on medical therapy. In general, the first goal of treatment is to relieve symptoms. When people first come to see a doctor and are diagnosed with Crohn's disease or ulcerative colitis, they are typically experiencing one or more symptoms of the disease. Knowing what is wrong and what is causing their symptoms is generally first and foremost in their mind, but close behind is the desire to get rid of the symptoms and feel healthy again.

Remission — the absence of symptoms — is obviously an important goal, and it is typically achieved by using a medication that controls inflammation in the intestine or suppresses the body's immune response. However, once the IBD patient's symptoms are controlled, it is important to prevent recurrence of the inflammation that can cause the symptoms to come back.

A recurrence of inflammation and symptoms is often called a flare. The second goal of IBD therapy is to prevent disease flares. Unfortunately, not all of the medications that effectively treat a flare will necessarily reduce the risk of a flare once a person's IBD is in remission, and none of the medications is 100% effective. Furthermore, there is strong evidence that, even when an IBD sufferer is in remission and has no symptoms, inflammation of the intestine often persists. This is particularly true in Crohn's disease.

In the past, doctors didn't really worry about the disconnect between how their patients were feeling and the inflammation they could see if they performed a colonoscopy or carried out an imaging study of the bowel. In some cases, their lack of concern was because the inflammation was fairly mild and they considered it to be not terribly important. However, there has been a shift in how we view the presence of bowel inflammation that is present even when a patient is feeling well and has no symptoms. We now believe that the presence of inflammation is a bad thing for a number of reasons:

1. The presence of inflammation in a patient who is in remission — that is, who has no symptoms — means that person has an increased risk of experiencing a disease flare and recurrence of symptoms, particularly if they are not on any form of therapy.

2. In Crohn's disease, the presence of bowel inflammation over many weeks, months, and years can, even in someone who has no symptoms, lead to irreversible bowel damage and complications such as narrowings (strictures), abscesses, and fistulas. These complications often require surgery to deal with them.

3. Although it appears that this type of irreversible bowel damage generally does not occur in individuals with

---

Response vs. Remission

When a patient notices an improvement in symptoms but the symptoms are not gone entirely, doctors call this a response to treatment. When a patient is feeling well or has no symptoms, or at most has minimal or mild symptoms, doctors call this being in remission.

ulcerative colitis, the presence of inflammation over many years increases the risk of colon cancer, and better control of inflammation may not only reduce the chance of a flare but may also reduce the risk of cancer.

For all of these reasons, there has been a move toward making elimination of active inflammation and healing of ulcers — called mucosal healing — a goal of therapy in IBD.

There are a number of challenges with setting mucosal healing as a goal of therapy. Mucosal healing is a higher hurdle to achieve than remission or elimination of symptoms, and therapies that effectively reduce inflammation and treat symptoms are not necessarily effective at healing mucosa, particularly in Crohn's disease. It may be that complete mucosal healing is an unrealistic goal even when effective therapies are used, particularly when someone has had Crohn's disease for many years. It is also important to consider that complete healing of all ulcers may not be necessary in order to avoid some of the complications of Crohn's disease.

Another challenge is that it can be difficult to establish whether mucosal healing has occurred; it is not as simple as determining whether a patient's symptoms have improved or gone away completely. Because blood tests and stool tests often do not provide sufficiently accurate information, a colonoscopy or imaging studies, or both, may be required to ascertain whether mucosal healing has occurred. This obviously means more inconvenience and discomfort for the patient, but if the information is important and will help to guide therapy that will, in turn, help improve the long-term prognosis, it is important to go to the trouble of getting those tests done.

Ideal Goals of Therapy

When it comes to treatment goals, immediate symptom control should be the first priority. But ultimately, the ideal goals of therapy are the long-term control of symptoms, avoidance of disease flares, and prevention of disease- and treatment-related complications. If these goals can be achieved, it should be possible for people with IBD to live a full life, with few or no limitations resulting from the disease or its treatment.

Medication Considerations

Making the decision to undergo drug treatment for IBD, as well as choosing what drug to take at what dose and for how long, can be very complicated. There is no standard treatment for IBD that is effective in all situations for all patients. Every patient and every situation is somewhat different. Decisions about medical therapy need to be tailored for each person to meet the nature of the disease, while taking into consideration personal circumstances. This typically involves consideration of the treatment goals, the chance of achieving those goals, and the possible side effects or risks of therapy. For some people in countries, states, or provinces where medication is not paid for through private or public health insurance plans, the cost of the medication may also be a consideration in making treatment decisions. Even in cases where medication is partially paid for by insurance plans, the cost to the patient may still be so high that it affects their decision on whether to take a particular drug.

Standard Treatments

The lack of a standard treatment for IBD is also due to the fact that IBD sufferers vary widely with respect to the form of IBD they have, the location within the gastrointestinal tract affected, the severity and aggressiveness of the disease, and the complications of the disease. Patients also vary widely with respect to the side effects they are willing to risk or able to tolerate. They may respond differently to the means of administering the drug — pills, liquid suspensions, injections under the skin, infusions into a vein, suppositories, or enemas. As a result, what might be the best treatment for one patient might not be the best treatment for another patient with the same disease severity, location, and complications. For some patients, surgery may be required; for others, symptoms can be treated with medications and surgery can be avoided.

Individualized Medication

The aggressiveness of the disease differs from patient to patient. Other differences depend on whether patients develop a complication of their disease, whether the disease location extends or becomes more widespread, and whether the inflammation becomes resistant to medical treatment.

Some patients with Crohn's disease have mild symptoms that respond extremely well to medical therapy and never progress to develop strictures, fistulas, or abscesses, whereas others seem to experience one or more of these complications within a matter of months or a few years. Once one of these complications has occurred, drug therapy is usually not effective at completely reversing the damage. In those instances, surgery is frequently required. Because these complications often require surgery, it would seem to be even more important to effectively treat Crohn's disease in these individuals before the disease progresses to that point.

Similarly, some patients with ulcerative colitis first present with inflammation that is limited to the rectum and sigmoid colon only, with the remainder of the large intestine being unaffected. In the majority of these patients, the disease remains localized to that last part of the large intestine, but a minority do have progression to involve all or most of the large intestine, a potentially more serious situation. When a patient is first diagnosed with IBD, it would be extremely helpful to know what the likely course of disease will

> ### Adapted Drugs
>
> The development of new drug therapies for IBD has, until recently, been quite slow and, in most instances, the medications that have been used in IBD have not been specifically developed for the treatment of IBD. Instead, they have been adapted from use in other disorders.

be. This will, in turn, help physicians make recommendations regarding the best therapy for a given patient and will help the patient and their family make the best decisions for their situation.

Step-Up or Top-Down Therapy

Clearly, if a given patient has a very good prognosis, with only a small chance of developing complications of disease or requiring surgery, it would be best to treat them first with medications that have a lower likelihood of side effects but may be somewhat less potent or consistent in terms of treating inflammation. If these medications are not effective in controlling inflammation and the associated symptoms of IBD, then they could be considered for the more potent therapies that may be associated with a higher chance of side effects.

- **Step-Up Therapy:** This is a stepwise approach to treatment based on response to the various available medications. It is still used in ulcerative colitis and has been the usual standard in patients with Crohn's disease.

  However, because of the potentially irreversible nature of the complications that can occur in Crohn's disease and the frequent need for surgery once they occur, there has been a move toward using the more potent and more consistently effective therapies that are more likely to result in ulcer healing earlier on in the course of the disease, before complications have occurred.

- **Top-Down Therapy:** Provided that treatments are effective and safe, readily available, and not excessively expensive, this approach would seem to be the best for many patients with Crohn's disease, particularly those who are likely to have a more aggressive or complicated disease course or who have more extensive involvement of the bowel from the time of first diagnosis.

Unfortunately, physicians cannot always predict which patients will have a more aggressive disease course, with complications and the need for surgery, and which patients will be unlikely to require surgery or have serious complications. Thus, it is not always easy to decide who might be a good candidate for top-down therapy. Although there are certain features of the disease and certain blood tests that might help with the determination, they are not sufficiently accurate to be reliable.

Drug Guidelines

A number of different medical groups and societies have developed guidelines for the treatment of IBD. However, these guidelines are only general recommendations based on the weight of evidence from clinical studies and from extensive personal experiences. They cannot reflect all of the subtleties and nuances of treatment in the individual patient and cannot be considered the standard treatment.

As a result, an alternative approach that is sometimes called accelerated step care has been developed. This is essentially step-up therapy, but it uses well-defined timelines and goals of therapy to assess the response to a given therapy. If those goals are not reached within a certain period of time, the next treatment is started. In this way, ineffective treatments are stopped and other treatments tried without leaving a patient on an ineffective treatment for a prolonged period.

Benefits vs. Risks Assessment

Any given person with IBD may be likely to respond positively to a given medication, but may not be willing to take the possible risk of certain rare serious side effects. Another person might be willing to accept a relatively high risk of side effects for the sake of receiving the most effective treatment. The final decision about medical treatment of IBD requires, under ideal conditions, a full discussion among the doctor, the patient, and, where necessary, the family.

In addition to nonsteroidal anti-inflammatory drugs, there are other medications that are thought to have the potential to cause exacerbations or flares of IBD. Many of these medications are available only by prescription from a doctor. Every time you are given a new prescription, ask your doctor what the effect of the new medication might be on your IBD and if it has any interaction with the other medications you might already be taking for your IBD. Your doctor may not have an answer right away but will consult a reference source or ask a colleague with more experience. With the hundreds and hundreds of available medications, it is very difficult for any one individual to know about all of the possible interactions or effects of all of the medications.

Personalized Medicine

The type of treatment approach based on individual patient prognosis or risk is often called personalized health care or personalized medicine. This is being touted as the best way to give the right therapy to the right patient at the right time so as to maximize the likelihood of beneficial short- and long-term effects while, at the same time, minimizing the risk of side effects or bad outcomes of treatment. On a societal level, this approach also ensures that the maximum benefit is achieved for the money spent on medical therapy for IBD by directing the most expensive treatments to the right patients based on their risk or prognosis.

Q **What are side effects?**

A Doctor and patient should assess the risks of drug therapy, not only the common and usually less serious side effects, but also the more rare and more serious potential side effects. Side effects can generally be divided into two categories – those that occur more often the higher the dose of the drug taken and those that are unpredictable and can occur at any dose of the drug. The first category of side effect may not occur in the majority of patients treated with the medication in the usual dose range, but tends to be more common the higher the dose used. These side effects can sometimes be dealt with by reducing the dose of the drug. The second category of side effects does not seem to occur more frequently at higher drug doses. These side effects appear to be similar to an allergic reaction and usually mean that the drug cannot be used anymore because the reaction may occur even at low doses.

Similar to the way that physicians are trying to develop risk profiles for IBD complications that can be used in individual patients, there has also been work done in developing risk profiles for an individual's likelihood of experiencing a given side effect to a given drug therapy. A small number of these predictive tests currently exist. For example, a blood test can predict the chance that a given patient will develop a serious but rare blood complication of treatment with azathioprine (Imuran) or 6-mercaptopurine (Purinethol). If this blood test shows a low level of an enzyme involved in the metabolism of these drugs, then a patient is at increased risk of this blood complication and, as a result, can develop serious and life-threatening infections. If this blood test is performed before starting treatment and is found to be abnormally low, these drugs will usually not be considered as viable options or, if they are used, they will be given at very low doses.

However, in most instances, there are no blood tests that will predict a high risk of side effects for most drugs used to treat IBD. As a result, doctors have to use other factors, such as a patient's age, to predict risk of side effects. It is clear that the risk of serious infection is higher in older patients treated with drugs that suppress the body's immune system as compared to younger individuals. This is why doctors are generally more reluctant to use immune-suppressant medications in elderly IBD patients. The higher risk of this particular serious side effect may begin to outweigh the possible benefit of treatment.

Doctor-Patient Consultation

Some patients will ask the doctor, "What do you think is best?" and then trust the doctor to make the final recommendation on their behalf, based on the doctor's knowledge and experience in treating IBD and any insight the doctor may have into the patient's individual circumstances and psychological makeup. Others may not be so compliant, finding that even an extensive discussion with the doctor about the treatment options is not sufficient. They will look for other sources of information, such as the Internet or other IBD patients, in order to try to make decisions for themselves. The reliability of these approaches to information gathering should be discussed with a health-care professional.

Drug Information Sources

Many physicians, clinics, and hospitals have printed sheets that outline the nature of the various medications used to treat IBD, including when they are to be used and what can be expected from their use, with information on how to recognize the possible side effects. Some pharmacies provide similar drug information sheets for patients at the time of drug dispensing. There are also some websites that offer similar drug information, but the quality of that information varies from site to site. If in doubt about the quality of the site and its information, check with your doctor.

Some medications also require specific monitoring with periodic blood tests, for example. The patient may need this information to make a treatment decision.

Whenever the treatment of IBD is discussed, the fact that it is a chronic and lifelong disorder must be considered. Although some medications may be very effective at controlling

Questions to Discuss with Your Doctor about Drug Therapy

- Is drug treatment of my IBD necessary?
- Is the treatment intended to bring a flare under control or is it intended to maintain a remission?
- What benefits can I expect from this treatment? What symptoms will improve and what symptoms are not likely to improve?
- How quickly can I expect to see an improvement?
- What type of follow-up is needed if I take this treatment?
- What are some of the common side effects?
- What are the serious side effects that can occur with this therapy?
- Are there any other options for drug therapy in my situation?
- What is the cost of treatment?
- How long will I have to be on this therapy?
- Is surgery a viable option in my situation? If it isn't, will this therapy reduce my future risk of needing surgery?

inflammation and symptoms for a short period of time — days or weeks — what is really needed are medications that can safely and effectively ensure that, once a disease flare is under control, the IBD sufferer will be less likely to experience a recurrence of disease flares. Ideally, these medications will not only reduce the likelihood of a disease flare but will also reduce the risk of disease complications and the need for surgery.

Drug Therapy Options

Recommendations for treatment are divided into broad categories. These categories are determined by two considerations: whether Crohn's disease or ulcerative colitis is being treated; and, within each disease, whether the aim is to bring a flare or symptoms of active disease under control or to keep a patient well once a remission has been obtained through whatever means necessary. In some instances, recommendations may be further subdivided according to the location of the disease within the gastrointestinal tract and the severity of a flare. Certain complications of the diseases, such as abscesses in Crohn's disease, may also be considered as belonging in another category of disease treatment. These categories may be important because, in the case of several medications, they appear to be effective only in very specific situations and not in other situations.

Each drug or category of drugs may be used for different indications within IBD. For example, antibiotics are typically not used in ulcerative colitis because they don't appear to be very effective, but in patients with Crohn's disease, antibiotics do appear to be effective and are often used to reduce pain, improve drainage, and reduce the risk of widespread infection when a complication, such as an abscess or fistula, has developed.

In recent years, several new medications have been tested and found to be effective for the treatment of ulcerative colitis and Crohn's disease. These therapies have been approved by regulatory authorities in many countries and are available to IBD sufferers in those countries. Almost certainly, additional treatments will be available in the coming years. Some of these new treatments will work in ways that are similar to existing treatments, and it is unlikely that they will offer significant advantages in terms of effectiveness. However, treatments that work differently from existing treatments may offer improvements in effectiveness and more options for people who have not responded to other treatments or for whom other treatments seem to have stopped working.

Having more treatment choices and more effective treatments available would seem to be a great advance for people with IBD. However, it has made decision-making about which treatment to take much more difficult and complicated. When offered three different treatment options, all of which are known to be effective for your particular form of IBD, you will almost certainly ask, "Is treatment A more effective than treatment B? Is treatment B more effective than treatment C? Is treatment C more effective than treatment A?" As more and more medications are considered, the number of questions will multiply.

Unfortunately, your physician probably won't have a firm answer to many of these questions because, in most instances, no studies have been done to directly compare the newer medications to one another. Although new medications are tested in rigorous clinical trials before they are approved for use in patients, they are often compared in those trials to older therapies or to placebo (no treatment). It is impossible, therefore, to determine for certain which of the newer treatments is the most effective. This makes decision-making for patients and physicians very difficult.

Often, it is other factors that help patients make the final decision. These factors may include how the medication is taken (in pill form by mouth, as a subcutaneous injection under the skin, as an intravenous injection into a vein, or as an enema or suppository into the rectum) and possible side effects that might occur. The cost of therapy may also influence the decisions about drug treatment. In some instances, a patient's insurance coverage may dictate which treatment they can receive, because insurers, who consider cost as a major factor in their decision about which drugs to cover, might not pay for all potential IBD treatments.

Who Decides?

We would like to think that the decision about treatment is made by patients, in consultation with their doctor, based on what is best for them. Unfortunately, other entities, such as insurance companies or government-run health plans — who may not have an individual's best interest as their primary motivation — are increasingly involved in treatment decision-making.

Nonsteroidal Anti-Inflammatory Drugs

In general, the class of medication that you should be most concerned about using is the nonsteroidal anti-inflammatory drugs (NSAIDs) used for pain relief, because they may result in disease flares in some people with IBD. These include drugs with the generic names diclofenac, sulindac, naproxen, and ibuprofen, to name a few. Although most are available only by prescription, naproxen and ibuprofen are available over the counter in the United States and Canada under many different brand names. Be sure to read labels on every over-the-counter medication you purchase, and if you're not certain about its impact on your condition, consult your pharmacist or doctor.

Pain Relief

Nonsteroidal anti-inflammatory drugs are commonly used to relieve pain and as an anti-inflammatory for a variety of forms of arthritis. Although not every IBD sufferer will run into problems when taking nonsteroidal anti-inflammatory drugs, a proportion find that they produce increased abdominal pain, diarrhea, and rectal bleeding. These drugs can be used in IBD patients if absolutely needed for the treatment of other forms of inflammation or sources of pain, but be certain that the indication for use is clear and that the treatment goals are equally clear so that therapy does not go on for any longer than necessary. Also consider other available alternatives that might be safer in IBD while achieving similar beneficial effects.

For relatively minor aches and pains, such as headaches, acetaminophen (Tylenol) is often effective and perfectly safe to take if you have IBD. If pain is more severe and an anti-inflammatory effect is not needed, then acetaminophen with codeine (for example Tylenol #2 or Tylenol #3) will provide pain relief without risk of causing a flare of the IBD.

Narcotics (Opioids)

Chronic use of codeine and other opioid medications, such as oxycodone (a component of Percocet and Percodan), meperidine (Demerol), or fentanyl, can lead to addiction. In IBD patients, these drugs should be used only for episodes of acute pain (for example, after surgery) where the cause of the pain is known and with a definite end point for completing therapy.

Pain Clinics

When someone with IBD has chronic pain that is not manageable through treatment of the underlying IBD or through simple nonspecific measures, such as acetaminophen, then referral to a chronic pain clinic is indicated. These clinics usually have a team made up of anesthetists (pain specialists), nurses, physiotherapists, occupational therapists, psychiatrists or psychologists, social workers, and pharmacists with the goal of controlling pain in individuals with chronic pain syndromes. In some cases, they may also employ alternative practitioners, such as acupuncturists.

Commonly Used IBD Medications

Mesalamine (5-Aminosalicylic Acid) Containing Preparations

- Sulfasalazine (Salazopyrin, Azulfidine)
- Delayed-release mesalamine (Asacol, Pentasa, Salofalk, Mezavant, Lialda)
- Balsalazide (Colazide)
- Olsalazine (Dipentum)

Glucocorticoids (Steroids)

- Prednisone
- Budesonide (Entocort, Cortiment, Uceris)
- Prednisolone
- Hydrocortisone
- Betamethasone (Betnesol)
- Methylprednisolone (Solu-Medrol)

Antibiotics

- Metronidazole (Flagyl)
- Ciprofloxacin (Cipro)

Immunosuppressants

- Azathioprine (Imuran)
- 6-mercaptopurine (Purinethol)
- Methotrexate
- Cyclosporine
- Tofacitinib (Xeljanz)

Biologic Therapies

- Infliximab (Remicade, Inflectra, Remsima)
- Adalimumab (Humira)
- Golimumab (Simponi)
- Certolizumab pegol (Cimzia)
- Vedolizumab (Entyvio)
- Ustekinumab (Stelara)

Mesalamine (5-Aminosalicylic Acid) Containing Drugs

Mesalamine (also known as 5-aminosalicylic acid or 5-ASA) has a chemical structure very similar to aspirin, but its medicinal properties are somewhat different. Unlike aspirin, 5-ASA is not a pain reliever, but it does appear to have many anti-inflammatory actions similar to aspirin, although its anti-inflammatory actions appear to be fairly specific to the intestinal tract. These anti-inflammatory activities in the intestinal tract are hoped for when medications containing 5-ASA are prescribed.

Taken as a pill or a powder, 5-ASA is very quickly absorbed from the upper part of the small intestine and it then enters into the bloodstream. However, for this drug to be effective, it has to be within the intestine and not in the bloodstream. Therefore, drugs containing 5-ASA that have been produced for IBD all have some way of keeping the 5-ASA within the intestine and preventing it from being absorbed before it gets down to the parts of the intestine most commonly affected by IBD.

Sulfasalazine

Sulfasalazine is composed of two parts — a sulfa antibiotic and 5-ASA — that are connected by a chemical bond. This bond is split by an enzyme produced by the bacteria present in the large intestine and the last part of the small intestine. This releases the sulfa antibiotic and the 5-ASA into the bowel, where they can act on the inflammation in the inner lining of the intestine. The beneficial action of sulfasalazine in IBD is primarily due to the 5-ASA part of the drug, although the whole intact drug, containing both sulfa and 5-ASA, may also have some beneficial effect.

When a flare of ulcerative colitis or Crohn's disease is severe, sulfasalazine and other 5-ASA-containing drugs are usually not effective. Trying to use them may end up having negative effects because of a possible delay in starting stronger or more effective medications. In those situations, the inflammation has probably progressed beyond a point where sulfasalazine can be effective.

Side Effects

In a small but significant proportion of patients, sulfasalazine was found to have a number of troubling side effects, most commonly stomach upset, often with nausea and vomiting, especially when higher doses were used. Unfortunately, higher doses appear to be more effective than lower doses that have fewer problems with stomach upset.

There are other side effects that can occur — skin rashes, fever, decreased blood cell counts, and infertility in males. Most of these occur only rarely and are not related to the dose of the medication, but they can be very severe. They appear to be due to the sulfa part of the drug. Knowing about this difference

Sulfasalazine Benefits

- Sulfasalazine medication is effective in treating the symptoms of ulcerative colitis as long as the inflammation in the colon isn't too severe. It also helps to keep the disease in remission once a flare has come under control.

- Sulfasalazine is probably effective in milder flares of Crohn's disease, but mainly when the large intestine is affected. However, it seems to be less effective when Crohn's disease affects the small intestine. Sulfasalazine also doesn't appear to prevent flares in Crohn's disease the way it does in ulcerative colitis.

in the impact of the two parts of the sulfasalazine molecule allowed researchers to develop newer 5-ASA-containing medications that do not have the sulfa associated with many of the side effects of sulfasalazine.

Controlled-Release Mesalamine (5-ASA) Preparations

To solve the problem of the side effects associated with the sulfa part of sulfasalazine and to prevent the 5-ASA part from being released and absorbed too far up in the small intestine, preparations have been formulated that keep the 5-ASA in the intestine and release it only when it gets to the area of the intestine where its maximum action is needed. This delay in the release of 5-ASA is achieved through several different means.

Some preparations of 5-ASA are coated in a waxy film that dissolves and releases the 5-ASA when the acid within the intestine becomes sufficiently neutralized. Examples of this type of preparation are Asacol, Pentasa, Salofalk, Mezavant, and Lialda. In Pentasa, the 5-ASA is present in hundreds of tiny granules within a tablet form designed to allow the 5-ASA to escape slowly over time as the tablet passes down through the small and large intestine.

Pentasa is also available in some countries as granules that can be mixed with fluids or food, thereby making them easier to ingest. The 5-ASA-containing preparations are typically taken between 2 and 4 times per day, but there is evidence that, in certain circumstances, the entire daily dose can be taken at once without causing any loss of beneficial effect and with no increase in side effects. This once-daily dosing is also effective with Mezavant, Lialda, and Asacol.

Side Effects

With the elimination of the sulfa part of the drug, the 5-ASA preparations result in fewer side effects, such as nausea, indigestion, and vomiting. Some of the other side effects occasionally experienced by patients taking sulfasalazine, such as the decreased blood count and infertility in males, also do not occur with the 5-ASA drugs. Patients receiving 5-ASA-containing preparations can still experience side effects, but they are usually mild.

Headaches

Patients occasionally find that they cannot take the higher doses required to treat IBD effectively because of headaches. At lower doses, patients usually find that headaches do not occur. Fortunately, most patients do not experience headaches, even

5-ASA Benefits

- The 5-ASA-containing drugs can usually be used at higher, more effective doses than sulfasalazine, enabling many patients to reach the higher doses required to treat their disease.

- The controlled-release 5-ASA medications are useful in milder flares of inflammatory bowel disease, particularly ulcerative colitis, and are helpful in reducing the risk of recurrent flares in patients with ulcerative colitis.

- When the 5-ASA drugs were first developed, it was hoped that they would provide a safe and effective alternative to steroid medications in patients with Crohn's disease. Unfortunately, they have not been found to be as effective in Crohn's disease as had been hoped for. Despite the fact that there is some controversy about their effectiveness in Crohn's disease, many physicians still elect to use 5-ASA drugs early in the course of the disease because of their excellent safety record.

- In some patients with Crohn's disease, particularly those with involvement of the large intestine and those with mild disease, the 5-ASA-containing drugs will sometimes produce a noticeable benefit without risking the side effects that might occur with the stronger drugs, such as prednisone or immunosuppressives. However, only a small minority of patients will respond to this treatment strategy, and it is important to ensure that 5-ASA treatment has resulted in reduced bowel inflammation and not just reduced symptoms.

- The 5-ASA drugs may also reduce the risk of recurrence of Crohn's disease following surgical removal of the affected segments of the intestine. They are particularly appealing in that situation when using a drug for a period of several years, because the 5-ASA drugs have a well-proven, long-term safety record.

at very high doses of 5-ASA. This is different from sulfasalazine, where many patients experience some type of side effect when a high dose is given.

Allergic Reactions
The allergic type of reactions that can occur unpredictably at any drug dose can occur as a result of 5-ASA use. These are extremely uncommon with 5-ASA, but can be very serious. Two examples of this type of side effect are pancreatitis (inflammation of the pancreas gland) and pericarditis (inflammation of the sac around the heart).

Convenience

Because 5-ASA is a relatively mild anti-inflammatory, high doses of the drug are required in order to see a beneficial effect. As a result, patients who are taking 5-ASA-containing compounds usually have to take multiple pills, sometimes in multiple doses. This is less convenient than other medications, which can be taken once per day or even once per week or once every few weeks.

Some of the companies that produce the 5-ASA-containing compounds have addressed this issue by making tablets that contain a large dose of the drug so that a fewer number of pills need to be taken. In addition, there is some evidence that these drugs may be able to be taken as little as twice per day or possibly even just once per day without losing the beneficial effect.

> **Long-Term Safety**
>
> The long-term safety of 5-ASA is excellent, with virtually no long-term side effects reported other than extremely rare damage to the kidney.

Balsalazide

Balsalazide (Colazide) is another drug in the 5-ASA category, similar to sulfasalazine, in that it contains 5-ASA chemically bonded to another molecule. This prevents the drug from being absorbed in the small intestine. When it reaches the large intestine, the 5-ASA is split from the carrier molecule by enzymes produced by bacteria in the large intestine, thereby allowing the 5-ASA to have its anti-inflammatory effect on the inner intestinal lining.

Side Effects

The possible side effects are similar to those of the 5-ASA-containing compounds.

Balsalazide Benefits

- Balsalazide is effective in treating mild flares of ulcerative colitis and in preventing relapses once the disease is in remission. It hasn't been tested adequately in Crohn's disease.
- High doses of balsalazide are usually well tolerated because the carrier molecule produces no significant side effects.

Olsalazine

Olsalazine (Dipentum) is composed of two 5-ASA molecules that are chemically bonded to each other. The two 5-ASA molecules cannot be absorbed effectively in the small intestine, but are split apart by the action of an enzyme produced by bacteria in the large intestine.

Olsalazine Benefits

- Olsalazine is effective in preventing relapses of ulcerative colitis once the disease is in remission.

Side Effects

Olsalazine is somewhat different from the other 5-ASA-containing drugs because in about 15% of people who take this medication, the two 5-ASA molecules bound together can irritate the lining of the small intestine, resulting in increased diarrhea. Obviously, this side effect can be confused with worsening of the IBD. Olsalazine can also produce the other side effects that are rarely seen with 5-ASA-containing drugs, but not any more commonly than is seen with the other 5-ASA preparations.

Mesalamine Enemas and Suppositories

In patients who have ulcerative colitis with the inflammation limited to the rectum and lower part of the large intestine, a very effective approach to treating the disease is to apply mesalamine (5-ASA) directly onto the inflamed intestinal lining by putting 5-ASA into an enema or a suppository. These types of enemas and suppositories are commercially available in many countries under a variety of brand names, such as Salofalk, Pentasa, Rowasa, Canasa, and Asacol.

Enemas

Most people think that an enema is used to treat severe constipation. Liquid (typically water) is put into the rectum and is expelled soon after with feces. However, medicated enemas containing 5-ASA are designed to be held in the rectum and the lower part of the large intestine so that the medication within the liquid has a chance to coat the intestinal lining and produce its beneficial effects.

Even when patients are willing to take a course of enema treatment, they may not be able to keep the enema in the rectum for long enough to allow it to be effective. This inability

Enema Option

While not an appealing prospect, most people will accept a course of enema treatment, especially if they know that it is more likely to make them better and to make them better more quickly than other approaches.

Mesalamine Enema and Suppository Benefits

- Mesalamine enemas or suppositories are considered to be the first choice of treatment for ulcerative colitis where the inflammation is limited to the rectum or to the lower part of the colon. These enemas or suppositories are more effective in that situation than the 5-ASA preparations taken by mouth.
- Mesalamine enemas and suppositories are also extremely safe, with virtually no risk of serious side effects.

to hold the enema usually occurs because the rectum is inflamed and, as a result, is very irritable and sensitive. When the rectum is irritable, there is typically a strong urge to empty the bowels as soon as there is something in the rectum causing it to be distended or stretched. This may be stool or it may be the liquid from the enema. The longer the enema is held, the

Steps for Administering an Enema

The mesalamine enema comes in a plastic bottle containing between 2 and 4 ounces (60 and 125 mL) of the medicated liquid. The bottle usually has a smooth, tapered tip that can be inserted into the anus, usually with the help of some lubricant or by moistening with water.

- Lubricate or moisten the anus.
- Lie on the left side with your knees tucked up toward your chest.
- Insert the tip of the bottle into the anus and squeeze the bottle so that the liquid is injected into the rectum and lower part of the colon. Try not to squeeze the entire contents of the bottle into the rectum too quickly.
- Stay on your left side for at least 15 minutes after taking the enema and, if possible, do not get up again after that. It is best if the enema can be kept in overnight, but this is not always possible for someone with active ulcerative colitis.
- If you have very severe inflammation of the rectum, you may begin to feel cramping and a strong urge to move your bowels soon after taking the enema. It may be possible to overcome this urge and cramping by lying still, taking deep breaths, and trying to relax.
- In some cases, the pressure and urgency may persist, preventing you from falling asleep. Ultimately, you may have to get up and move your bowels.
- If you cannot retain the enema overnight, then keeping it in for at least 1 to 2 hours should still provide some benefit.

farther up the colon it tends to spread and coat the surface. In general, most enemas do not reach much above the sigmoid colon and, as a result, are not fully effective for half or more of patients with ulcerative colitis.

Enemas are usually prescribed to be taken once per day, in the evening, as the last thing you do before going to sleep. This helps to ensure that the enema is held in the rectum and colon as long as possible. Many patients with IBD are able to administer an enema themselves, but some do require assistance because it requires flexibility to insert the tip of the enema bottle or tubing into the anus.

Suppositories

Some people who cannot tolerate or retain enemas are able to keep a 5-ASA-containing suppository in the rectum long enough for it to have an effect. The suppository usually dissolves very quickly and leaves only a thick pasty material containing the medication. Suppositories are large capsules or tablets with one end rounded and tapered, which allows the suppository to be inserted through the anus into the rectum, where the suppository dissolves, releasing the active medication.

Suppositories should be taken at bedtime, although some doctors advocate taking them twice daily, in the morning and at bedtime, to improve effectiveness. Despite this, most studies show that one nighttime dose every day is equally as effective.

Glucocorticoid (Steroid) Medications

When a doctor has an IBD patient with very active or severe disease, steroids have traditionally been the drugs prescribed. There are a number of steroids available on the market, and although they have slightly different chemical forms, they all have similar actions in IBD, with the exception of budesonide.

Steroids have been used for many decades in the treatment of inflammatory bowel disease. For most of this time, they have been the most consistently effective class of medications, having the advantage over many other classes of treatment because they generally work very quickly and can be used in a wide variety of forms of IBD.

The steroid medications used to treat IBD should not be confused with the steroids that are often talked about and still sometimes used for enhancing performance in athletes or body builders — the anabolic steroids. In fact, the steroids used to

Oral Steroid Benefits and Drawbacks

- Oral steroids, such as prednisone, typically begin working very quickly. In many instances, patients begin to feel better within several days of starting treatment, although complete disappearance of symptoms may take several weeks. This rapid action is a very attractive property of steroids, differentiating them from several other classes of medications, such as 5-ASA, that tend to take significantly longer to take effect.

- Although steroids are generally quite effective for the treatment of IBD, they have two main drawbacks — their lack of benefit when used to prevent recurrence of disease flares once the disease has been brought into remission, and their potential for producing short-term and long-term side effects. Some of these side effects may not reverse or go away once the dose is reduced or stopped.

treat IBD have the opposite effect, if taken for long periods, of causing a loss of muscle bulk and strength.

Oral Steroids (Prednisone)

The most commonly prescribed oral steroid in North America is prednisone. It is inexpensive, typically costing only a few cents per day, and very effective, but has the risk of serious side effects, some of which can be very troubling and, in some cases, irreversible. Approximately half of patients who take steroids experience at least one side effect. For most of those patients, the side effects are not severe, but there is a significant minority who find the experience of being on steroids so negative that it makes them decide to never take steroids again, no matter how bad their IBD gets.

Dosage Regimen

When taken in oral form, steroids can usually be taken once per day, typically in the morning. They do not necessarily have to be taken with meals, although this may reduce some of the potential for indigestion that some patients experience while taking higher doses of the drugs. Steroids are usually taken in courses of treatment lasting from 2 to 4 months.

Patients with an acute flare of IBD are usually started on a relatively high dose — 40 to 60 mg of prednisone per day — and the dose is gradually tapered over a period of 2 to 4 months. Different doctors may recommend different tapering schedules, and there is no evidence that one approach is better or worse than another.

Cold Turkey

Prednisone must not be stopped suddenly, or "cold turkey," once it has been taken for more than 10 to 14 days. You may experience feelings of weakness, light-headedness, muscle and joint pain, abdominal pain, and diarrhea if you stop prednisone too quickly.

Q **What is steroid dependency?**

A Although studies have shown that prednisone is not nearly as effective at preventing flares as it is at treating flares, many patients who are started on prednisone are not able to get off it for many months or, in some cases, even years. These people are what doctors refer to as "steroid dependent." This doesn't mean that they have an addiction to the medication. Rather, when the dose of prednisone is gradually reduced after controlling a flare, the disease worsens and the patient has to increase the dose again.

Some IBD patients who have difficulty coming off steroids find that stopping or reducing the dose makes them feel bad – what they describe as the "blahs." They feel tired and weak and may lose their appetite. This is not due to a flare of active IBD; rather, the adrenal glands are not producing natural steroids because this process has been suppressed by the long-term use of prednisone or other steroid medication.

When steroid medication is suddenly stopped and the adrenal glands cannot produce their own steroids, a patient can become very ill and even go into shock. This can usually be avoided by slowly reducing the dose of prednisone over many weeks or months. Directions from a physician on how to reduce the dose and discontinue prednisone is very important.

However, prednisone and other steroids should not be stopped suddenly once they have been taken for a period of more than 10 to 14 days. Although this type of slow tapering of prednisone may reduce the chance that the IBD flares again as the dose is reduced, it is probably just as important in preventing the symptoms of steroid withdrawal.

Common and Reversible Side Effects
The most common side effects of prednisone affect a person's appearance, including increased appetite and weight gain, swelling of the feet and hands, rounding of the face (so-called moon face), acne, and easy bruising. For people who are very concerned about their appearance or who depend upon their appearance for their livelihood, these may be unacceptable side effects.

Fortunately, these common side effects tend to go away as a person reduces the dose of prednisone and is able to discontinue it. However, it typically takes much longer for the effects to go away as compared with how quickly they may begin as a person starts taking prednisone.

Weight Gain
The weight gain often seen with prednisone treatment may also seem like a positive effect for patients with IBD, who often

have problems with weight loss or keeping weight on. However, the weight gain that occurs in patients taking steroids is not a healthy type of weight gain. Most of the weight that is gained on steroids tends to be due to an increase in fatty tissue rather than an increase in muscle or lean body mass. This increase in body fat may take quite some time — usually many months — to come off once a person stops taking steroids.

Mood Swings and Sleep Disturbances

Another side effect that may be very troubling to patients is the mood swings and sleep disturbance that may come with high doses of prednisone (usually 40 mg per day or more). Some patients describe feeling "high" or "energized" while on prednisone, and many find it very difficult to fall asleep and stay asleep. Although this may seem like a positive effect for some people, in the long term it can lead to increasing fatigue, diminished work or school performance, and even psychiatric disturbances.

Depression

Steroids may also lead to depression, particularly in people who have a prior history of depression before going on the medication.

Sleep Problems

The sleep problems can be minimized by taking the dose of steroids in the morning, although when the problem is severe, this may not help very much and sleeping pills are often not effective. In many cases, the only solution is reducing the dose and stopping the steroids.

Steroid Side Effects

Common and Reversible

- Rounding of the face (moon face)
- Acne
- Weight gain
- Fluid retention (e.g., swelling of feet and hands)
- Increased appetite
- Insomnia and sleep disturbance
- Easy bruising and poor wound healing
- Mood swings
- Increased energy

Uncommon and Possibly Irreversible

- High blood pressure
- Diabetes
- Cataracts
- Osteoporosis
- Increased pressure inside the brain
- Thinning of the skin
- Impaired wound healing
- Increased susceptibility to certain infections
- Avascular necrosis of hip or other joint

Calcium Supplements

For patients who have normal bone density when they start on steroids, there is no single accepted way to reduce the risk of bone loss due to steroids. At a minimum, you should ensure adequate intake of calcium and vitamin D and, if it is not adequate, take supplementation. Dairy products are usually the main source of calcium, but many IBD patients avoid them. In those individuals, supplementation is very important.

Uncommon and Possibly Irreversible Side Effects

Fortunately, most of the side effects described earlier tend to go away as the dose of steroid is decreased or after the steroid is stopped altogether. However, there are a number of side effects that tend to occur when steroids are used chronically, for many months or years, or that tend to be irreversible and do not go away even after steroids are stopped. Some of these are very rare and unpredictable, whereas the risk of others seems to increase the longer steroids are used.

These side effects include loss of bone strength or density (osteoporosis), clouding of the lens in the eyes (cataracts), increased blood pressure, increased blood sugar (diabetes), increased pressure inside the brain, thinning of the skin, impaired healing of wounds or cuts, and increased susceptibility to certain types of infections. Some of these complications, such as cataracts, are irreversible, whereas others, such as high blood pressure, high blood sugar, poor wound healing, and increased risk of infections, may diminish in severity or go away entirely when steroids are tapered and stopped. There is currently no way to predict the occurrence of these side effects, but they tend to occur more often the higher the dose and the longer the use.

Hypertension and Diabetes

Steroids are more likely to cause an increase in blood pressure or blood sugar in someone who is already predisposed or at risk of developing hypertension (high blood pressure) or diabetes (high blood sugar), respectively. Although steroids can be used in people with hypertension or diabetes, special care and close monitoring is required and, in many cases, alternative medications are tried before considering the use of steroids.

Osteoporosis

The loss of bone density (osteoporosis) is something that tends to occur relatively slowly, although more rapid bone loss can occur in the first few months of steroid treatment. The use of a special X-ray called dual energy X-ray absorptiometry (DEXA) is a safe and accurate way of measuring bone density over time.

In IBD patients who already have reduced bone density when they are started on steroids, the use of bisphosphonates (etidronate, alendronate, and risedronate) is frequently recommended. These drugs are most effective when taken along with calcium supplements, and can sometimes result in an increase in bone density. This usually requires a specific schedule of bisphosphonate and calcium dosing, with careful monitoring by a doctor.

These particular bisphosphonates are taken in pill form by mouth and can produce irritation of the gastrointestinal system and associated symptoms, such as abdominal pain and diarrhea. This can make it difficult for some IBD patients to take these medications. However, there are some bisphosphonates, such as pamidronate, zoledronate, and ibandronate, that can be administered intravenously on a relatively infrequent basis — anywhere from once every 3 months to once per year — and do not cause gastrointestinal symptoms.

Avascular Necrosis

One particular complication of steroid treatment that is particularly feared is avascular necrosis. This is a very rare and unpredictable condition that can occur without warning even after a relatively short course of steroid treatment. Avascular necrosis involves a loss of the normal blood flow to the end of a bone, resulting in collapse of the end of the bone, which leads to pain and chronic arthritis. It most commonly affects the hips, but can occur in many other joints, including the knees and shoulders. The risk of this complication occurring in someone receiving prednisone is very small — much less than 1 chance in 100. What makes the situation even more complicated is the fact that it appears that avascular necrosis can, in rare instances, be a result of the underlying IBD rather than steroid treatment.

There is no known way of predicting who might develop avascular necrosis, but there has been some suggestion from experts that treatment with bisphosphonates may reduce the risk of avascular necrosis.

MRI is probably the best test to diagnose avascular necrosis. When detected early, before collapse of the bone has occurred, avascular necrosis of the hip can be treated by a surgical procedure called a core decompression. This procedure involves putting a hole in the outer lining of the bone to allow the increased pressure present in the center of the bone to be released and normal blood flow to resume.

Intravenous Steroids

Although most steroid treatment in IBD is given as prednisone in a pill taken by mouth, steroids can also be given as an infusion into the vein (intravenous) in patients who are very sick with IBD and who require hospital admission for close monitoring and possible treatment of complications.

Hospitalized patients whose IBD flare comes under control with intravenous steroids will typically be switched over to prednisone taken by mouth shortly before they are ready to be

Reducing Risk

Any unusual joint pain, particularly in the hips, in someone receiving steroids for IBD should be taken seriously and be investigated. Early detection of avascular necrosis in the hip through the use of X-rays, bone scans, or MRI (magnetic resonance imaging) may reduce risk of collapse of the bone and arthritis.

Pregnancy and Steroids

Steroid therapies such as prednisone can generally be used in pregnancy and are frequently used when a severe flare of IBD occurs during pregnancy. However, there does appear to be a slight increased risk of cleft lip or cleft palate if steroids are used in the late first trimester and the second trimester.

discharged from hospital. Usually, they are put on a relatively high dose of prednisone — somewhere in the range of 50 to 60 mg per day — and the dose is gradually reduced over a period of 2 to 4 months.

Rescue Therapy

Several medical "rescue therapies" for patients not responding to a 5- to 10-day course of intravenous steroid therapy have been advocated as effective ways of avoiding surgery. Among these rescue drugs are cyclosporine and infliximab. It may be possible to predict which patients will not respond to the standard intravenous steroid treatment and to treat them early with rescue therapy rather than waiting 5 to 10 days. This may result in better outcomes and may reduce some of the possible side effects of extended treatment with steroids. Some patients with severe IBD flares who do not respond to intravenous steroids do not want to consider the use of "rescue therapy" and may opt instead for surgery as the most effective way of dealing with the acute problem.

Budesonide

Unlike other steroids given in a pill or capsule form and taken by mouth, budesonide is very quickly broken down into a by-product that has no side effects once it is absorbed from the intestine into the bloodstream. Unfortunately, that by-product is also ineffective at treating IBD. There are, however, two forms of oral budesonide available to treat IBD, Entocort and Uceris (known as Cortiment MMX in Canada), that are encased in a special formulation that prevents the budesonide from being absorbed into the bloodstream and releases it only when it reaches the part of the intestine that is inflamed. The budesonide then acts on the inner surface of the intestine to reduce inflammation and treat symptoms of IBD. Entocort is designed to release the budesonide in the last part of the small intestine (the ileum) and the first part of the colon (ascending colon), so it is used to treat Crohn's disease, which often involves those areas. Uceris, or Cortiment MMX, is designed to release the budesonide throughout the entire colon, so it is used to treat ulcerative colitis.

Budesonide is also available in some countries in an enema form for the treatment of ulcerative colitis affecting the lower part of the colon and rectum.

Side Effects

Side effects can occur, particularly with higher doses taken for prolonged periods. The typical dose is 9 mg per day given as one dose, usually in the morning. Like conventional steroids, budesonide does not seem to be highly effective at keeping Crohn's disease patients in remission once the acute flare has been brought under control, although some patients who respond to the acute treatment seem to remain well when kept on a slightly lower dose of 6 mg per day. For ulcerative colitis patients, it is still not clear whether continuing budesonide once the acute flare is under control is an effective and safe way of reducing the chance of another flare.

Keep in mind that budesonide is a steroid and monitoring for complications and side effects, such as loss of bone density, is still necessary.

Budesonide Benefits

- When released, budesonide has a local effect on the inner lining of the intestine and results in decreased inflammation and improved symptoms. Any portion of the drug absorbed into the bloodstream then gets inactivated and side effects are unlikely to occur.
- Budesonide is effective at treating mild flares of Crohn's disease involving the ileum and mild or moderate flares of ulcerative colitis with much less risk of side effects than "conventional" steroids, such as prednisone.

Steroid Enemas and Suppositories

There are a number of different commercially available medicated enemas and suppositories that contain steroids. The most commonly used steroid for enemas is hydrocortisone (Hycort, Cortenema). As with 5-ASA, steroids can be formulated into suppositories to treat ulcerative proctitis (ulcerative colitis affecting only the rectum). In some countries, steroid foam enemas (Cortifoam) are available. These can have an advantage over standard liquid enemas that is similar to the advantages of suppositories — they are easier to hold in the rectum for some people who cannot hold the liquid enemas.

Side Effects

Some patients who respond to steroid enemas need to keep taking them to keep the disease under control. In those instances, with particular steroids, such as betamethasone (Betnesol), it is possible to start seeing more of the common steroid side effects, such as acne, water retention, and weight gain.

Naveen is 19 years old and is studying environmental landscape management at a local community college. He lives with his parents and his younger brother and sister. His brother was diagnosed with Crohn's disease at the age of 12 and had surgery within 2 years of his diagnosis. Fortunately, he has done well since surgery.

For the past 2 months, Naveen has occasionally been noticing some blood in his stools and some pain and swollen lumps around his anus when he wipes after a bowel movement. He has also been feeling a bit "off" and is not as energetic as usual. He has had some mild cramping in the abdomen, and diarrhea from time to time. He has lost about 15 pounds (7 kg) even though his food intake has not changed. His parents are concerned that he, too, might have Crohn's disease, and they convince him to go to see their family doctor.

The family doctor listens to his story and orders blood tests, stool tests, and an ultrasound of his abdomen. Like Naveen's parents, the doctor is concerned that he may be showing signs of Crohn's disease. Rather than waiting for the results of the tests, he immediately refers Naveen to a gastroenterologist for a consultation. The family doctor calls the gastroenterologist and relays his concerns about Naveen, and she arranges for a consultation with Naveen within 2 weeks.

By the time the gastroenterologist sees Naveen, the results of his tests have come back. The blood tests reveal that he is quite anemic and has low iron levels. His blood C-reactive protein level, a marker of inflammation, is elevated, and the ultrasound shows a segment of thickened small intestine that appears to be inflamed. She concludes that it is almost certain that Naveen has Crohn's disease, but she needs some additional tests to confirm the diagnosis and determine the full extent of the disease. She arranges to carry out a colonoscopy and an MRI scan of the small intestine (MR enterography).

The colonoscopy reveals some inflammation and ulcers at the bottom of the rectum. The rest of the large intestine (colon) is normal, but there is inflammation and some large ulcers in the short segment of small intestine that she is able to see during the colonoscopy. The doctor also sees that there are swollen skin tags around the outside of the anus. These are probably what Naveen has been feeling in that area.

The doctor is now quite certain that Naveen has Crohn's disease and discusses several treatment options with him. She suggests that, while they wait for the biopsy results and the MRI scan, he start on prednisone. She also recommends that he see his family doctor and make sure that his immunizations are up to date, because it is likely he is going to need medications that suppress his immune system…

(continued on page 193)

Steroid Enema and Suppository Benefits

- Steroid enemas are generally indicated for the treatment of active ulcerative colitis of the rectum and lower part of the colon, but are sometimes used for the treatment of Crohn's disease involving the rectum. Although steroid enemas are effective in ulcerative colitis, they are typically used in instances where 5-ASA (mesalamine) enemas have been tried and have been found to not be effective.

- Steroid enemas have an advantage over oral or intravenous forms of steroids because patients taking steroid enemas do not commonly experience significant side effects, for at least two reasons. First, the amount of steroid medication in the enema is generally much less than the amount taken when the disease is treated with medication taken by mouth. This lower dose may be effective because the drug is put directly on the affected area of intestine rather than acting indirectly after being absorbed from the upper small intestine into the bloodstream. Second, the drug in the enema may not be well absorbed through the lining of the rectum or colon and, as a result, will not have any effect throughout the body. The amount of steroid in the various enemas and the amount that gets absorbed into the bloodstream do vary quite a bit from enema to enema.

- In addition to being used to treat ulcerative colitis of the rectum and lower part of the colon, suppositories and enemas can be used in combination with oral 5-ASA or steroids. They can sometimes be helpful in reducing the inflammation that is present in the rectum more quickly than oral medication. This may be greatly appreciated by patients because the symptoms they experience from inflammation of the rectum (urgency to move the bowels, loss of control, a feeling of incomplete emptying after a bowel movement, and pain in the rectum) are some of the most troubling they may experience.

Antibiotics

Some antibiotics appear to benefit patients with Crohn's disease, especially the antibiotic metronidazole (Flagyl). The next most commonly used antibiotic in Crohn's disease is ciprofloxacin (Cipro).

When antibiotics are used to treat infections, it is important that the indication for antibiotic use is clear. Antibiotics are active only against bacteria and are not needed for viral infections, such as colds or flus. They should not be prescribed unless there is a strong suspicion or confirmation of a bacterial infection.

In particular, antibiotics appear to be useful in Crohn's disease when the large intestine is involved or when complications, such as abscesses or fistulas, have occurred.

Antibiotics are not usually used for long-term maintenance treatment, but some patients have recurrent symptoms when antibiotics are stopped and seem to fare better if they are kept on continuous long-term antibiotic therapy, sometimes in relatively low doses.

Antibiotic Benefits

- Although the effectiveness of antibiotics in IBD is not proven or accepted by all doctors, most do believe that antibiotics are effective in selected individuals with Crohn's disease and possibly also some with ulcerative colitis.

Antibiotics for Other Illnesses

There is a common misconception that antibiotics taken for reasons other than treating IBD can actually cause flares of IBD. While this may not be true, it is important that patients with IBD take antibiotics only for very clear indications, because the use of most antibiotics can lead to an intestinal infection with a bacteria called *Clostridium difficile*. This infection can occur in people without IBD, but in someone with IBD, it can present a lot like an IBD flare, with a lot of watery diarrhea. A *Clostridium difficile* infection in an IBD patient can make the IBD very difficult to treat or can lead to a flare of the underlying IBD.

Side Effects

While antibiotics generally do not cause flares of IBD, there are certain side effects that can occur when using antibiotics to treat IBD.

Metronidazole

Metronidazole (Flagyl) can produce an effect on the nerves in the hands and feet, leading to a sensation of numbness and tingling. If severe, this can lead to muscle weakness. If patients taking Flagyl drink alcohol, they might feel very bad and experience a reaction that may include weakness, sweating, and flushing. Flagyl appears to be safe to use during pregnancy, particularly when used for only a short course of 7 days.

Most of the side effects are seen more frequently when higher doses are used; accordingly, there has been a tendency away from prescribing high doses of metronidazole. Ciprofloxacin has been used in combination with metronidazole by many doctors. When ciprofloxacin is added to metronidazole, the dose of metronidazole can often be reduced so that the side effects are less likely to occur.

Ciprofloxacin

Ciprofloxacin is usually well tolerated and has very few obvious side effects. The most common is an increase in the amount of diarrhea, which is usually temporary and tends to decrease as the ciprofloxacin produces improvement in the disease. There are some concerns about women taking ciprofloxacin during pregnancy because of possible effects on cartilage and joint development in the fetus. For similar reasons, ciprofloxacin has usually been avoided in children.

> **Yeast Infections**
>
> Vaginal yeast infections are a common side effect that may occur in women taking antibiotics, particularly if the antibiotics are taken for more than 1 to 2 weeks. This may not go away with the usual medications to treat yeast infections until after the antibiotics have been stopped.

Immunosuppressant Medications

Immunosuppressant medications cause some suppression of the body's immune response, which may be beneficial in IBD because the disease involves overactivity or over-response of the body's immune system to something in the body or in the surrounding environment. The immunosuppressant medications used most commonly to treat IBD are azathioprine, 6-mercaptopurine, methotrexate, and cyclosporine.

In order to be useful, immunosuppressant medications must be used within a very narrow range of immune suppression so that patients do not become overly susceptible to infections. Even when used in appropriate doses, these drugs do increase the risk of certain types of infections, usually to a small extent, which varies from drug to drug.

Azathioprine and 6-Mercaptopurine

The value of azathioprine (Imuran) and 6-mercaptopurine (Purinethol) in treating IBD has been recognized since they were first used in the 1960s and 1970s. Although they are different drugs, they work in the same way and are considered to be interchangeable. Azathioprine and 6-mercaptopurine (6-MP) are given in pill form, taken once a day.

Azathioprine and 6-Mercaptopurine Benefits

- Azathioprine and 6-mercaptopurine are useful for keeping patients in remission and reducing the need, over time, for other medications, such as steroids.

- The effectiveness of these drugs in Crohn's disease is generally well accepted, but they have also been used in ulcerative colitis, where their usefulness is more controversial.

- They appear to be safe for children, in whom they are used in order to avoid the need for repeated courses of steroids. However, there has been some concern about increased risk of a rare form of cancer of the lymph glands (lymphoma) in young males; as a result, many doctors have been using other types of therapy for those patients.

- There are reports of many women who have taken azathioprine or 6-MP during pregnancy without any bad effects on either the course of the pregnancy or on the baby. However, it is still not possible to completely prove that these drugs are safe in pregnancy, and any consideration of using them during pregnancy requires a careful and complete discussion between a woman and her doctor about the risks of continuing and the risks of stopping the medication.

- Azathioprine has also been found to be effective in Crohn's disease when used in combination with one of the newer biologic drugs, infliximab (Remicade). When used in people who have not had Crohn's disease very long and have not been previously treated with immune suppressants, the combination of azathioprine and infliximab is more effective than either drug given alone. Whether this benefit of combination therapy extends to the use of other biologic drugs, such as adalimumab (Humira), has not been specifically tested. In ulcerative colitis, it appears that the combination of azathioprine and infliximab may offer an advantage over either therapy alone, but this is far from settled.

Long-Term Treatment

Azathioprine and 6-mercaptopurine are very slow-acting medications with respect to their beneficial effects. Once they are started, it usually takes 3 months on average for them to take full effect. As a result, they are not useful for treating acute flares of IBD, since most patients who are experiencing symptoms of active disease cannot wait for 3 months for their symptoms to improve.

When an IBD sufferer is started on azathioprine or 6-MP, it is usually with the understanding that it is a long-term treatment strategy — typically 3 or 4 years or more. Knowing whether or when to stop azathioprine or 6-MP in individuals who have responded well to them is extremely difficult. Most experts suggest that a minimum of 4 years is required before stopping therapy in someone who has done well. However, if there have been minor flares despite azathioprine or 6-MP therapy, it is likely that more severe flares will occur if the drug is stopped even after 4 years or more of therapy.

Side Effects

Although they require ongoing monitoring of blood tests, azathioprine and 6-MP are generally very well tolerated. A very small number of people experience nausea or gastrointestinal upset, but most patients experience no side effects that would make them aware that they are even taking medication. There are rare serious complications, however.

Allergies

Allergic reactions can occur, showing up as fever, skin rash, and worsening of IBD symptoms.

Abnormal Liver Blood Tests

Abnormal liver blood tests can also occur. Most often this does not occur with any symptoms and, as a result, requires monitoring of blood tests to detect. These abnormalities may be due to inherited differences among people in the way these drugs are metabolized and may improve with changes in drug dose. Liver blood test abnormalities may also be related to allergic reactions.

Pancreatitis

Azathioprine and 6-MP can result in pancreatitis (inflammation of the pancreas) in approximately 3% of patients receiving the medications. This is a potentially serious side effect that frequently requires hospitalization. In general, if pancreatitis does not occur in the first few weeks of treatment, it does not occur at all. If it does occur, it means that azathioprine or 6-MP cannot be used again for that individual.

Infection and Bleeding Complications

The dose of azathioprine or 6-MP initially prescribed for an individual patient is calculated based on the patient's weight. However, because of the differences in drug metabolism from person to person, the dose may have to be modified based on blood testing. When the dose of drug is too high for a given individual, the bone marrow's production of white blood cells (cells that help fight infection) and platelets (cells that are important in blood clotting) may decrease, leading to an increased risk of serious infection or bleeding complications.

Monitoring

Ongoing monitoring of blood tests is required as long as someone is taking azathioprine or 6-mercaptopurine. Initially, this may be as frequently as once per week, but for patients who have been on a stable dose without any abnormalities on blood testing, they can probably be checked once every 2 to 3 months. The ongoing monitoring is necessary because abnormalities can happen after many months or even years of being stable on the medication.

If the levels of these cells get too low, the dose of the drug usually needs to be reduced or, in some cases, the drug must be stopped. Measuring the numbers of white blood cells and platelets in the blood is an easy and inexpensive way of monitoring the effect of azathioprine and 6-MP on the bone marrow. However, they are only indirect measurements of how much of the active by-product of the drugs reaches the bloodstream. More recently, other blood tests have been developed to directly measure the level of the active drug by-products in the bloodstream. This may allow more precise monitoring of drug dosing, but it has not yet been adopted into routine practice by most doctors.

Thiopurine Methyltransferase Enzyme

There is a blood test that measures thiopurine methyl-transferase (TPMT), a key enzyme that determines how much of the active by-product is made for a given dose of the drug. This enzyme is abnormal or absent in a very small proportion of people (approximately 1 out of every 300 people). People who are lacking this enzyme produce very high levels of the active by-product and are at risk of developing severe reductions in white blood cells and platelets.

If patients are tested for this enzyme and found not to have it, they should probably not be treated with azathioprine or 6-MP or should be treated with very low doses. This blood test is still not used by many doctors because it is not widely available. What is often done instead is that the drug is started at approximately half of the dose that is calculated likely to be needed, and the white blood cell count and platelet count are closely followed for several weeks. If there is no sudden drop in the counts, the dose is then increased up to the target dose and the blood tests are continued to be followed closely.

Even if the white blood cell count remains normal for the first months after a person is started on azathioprine or 6-MP, a drop in the count can occur at any time during treatment. Although the risk is much lower than during the first few months, ongoing checking of blood tests is necessary as long as the person is taking the medication.

Cancer Risk

One of the most difficult issues for patients and doctors when considering the use of immunosuppressants, such as azathioprine and 6-MP, is the potential for future development of cancer. Any time there is suppression of the immune response, there is a theoretical increase in the risk of developing cancer. This has been extensively examined in patients who have been treated with azathioprine and 6-MP. Overall, it appears that the use of these drugs in IBD does not increase the risk of most forms of cancer, with the possible exceptions of lymphoma (a rare form of cancer of the lymph glands), certain forms of skin cancer, and cancer of the cervix.

Although nothing can be done to prevent or monitor for lymphoma, there are ways in which IBD patients can reduce their risk of skin cancer or cervical cancer. For prevention of skin cancer, avoiding sun exposure or protecting against sunburns with clothing or high-SPF sunscreens is very effective. It is also important that any unusual, new, changing, or enlarging skin lesions be checked out by a doctor. For cancer of the cervix, vaccination against the human papillomavirus (HPV) reduces the risk, and regular Pap testing will help pick up early treatable lesions before they develop into cancer.

Not a Cure
Although these drugs may be effective at controlling disease symptoms over many months or even years, they are not cures for IBD. When treatment is stopped, the disease can recur and flare up with symptoms coming back, sometimes worse than prior to first starting immune suppression therapy. As a result, many doctors are reluctant to stop treatment in someone who is doing well, even when it has been more than 4 years. Certainly, if there has been any sign of ongoing inflammation despite the fact that a person has had no significant symptoms, it is probably not wise to consider stopping therapy.

Methotrexate
Methotrexate was originally used to treat certain types of cancers. It interferes with the production of the genetic material, DNA, which, in turn, reduces the formation of new immune reactive cells, resulting in immunosuppression. Methotrexate may also have some anti-inflammatory action that may make it even more beneficial in IBD.

Now, methotrexate is used much more commonly in the treatment of chronic inflammatory disorders, such as rheumatoid arthritis or Crohn's disease, than in the treatment of cancer. To treat inflammatory disorders, methotrexate is usually taken once per week, either by mouth or by injection under the skin or into a muscle.

Side Effects
Methotrexate is usually well tolerated, although some people experience nausea and sometimes vomiting. This typically occurs on the day of the week when the methotrexate is taken. This side effect can usually be avoided or reduced by taking the

Minimal Risk

Minimal Risk

Although the use of azathioprine or 6-MP may increase the risk of lymphoma, the risk to any given individual taking these medications is extremely small. It has been calculated that azathioprine would need to be taken for more than 4,300 years for someone between the ages of 20 and 29 before observing one extra case of lymphoma. The risk of most other cancers is not different in people taking azathioprine or 6-MP than in individuals not taking one of these drugs.

Methotrexate Benefits

- Methotrexate is used in many of the same situations as azathioprine and 6-MP.
- It is effective in treating active Crohn's disease that has not adequately responded to steroids, such as prednisone, and, once the disease has been brought under control, is helpful in keeping the disease in remission and avoiding repeated treatments with steroids.
- It is not clear whether methotrexate is effective in ulcerative colitis.
- In patients with rheumatoid arthritis, methotrexate is often given in combination with biologic drugs, such as infliximab (Remicade), where it has been consistently shown to increase the effectiveness of these drugs. This same strategy has not been shown to be effective in IBD, although the use of methotrexate does seem to lower the amount of antibodies that form against infliximab. These antibodies are potentially important because they can increase the possibility of side effects from infliximab and may reduce its effectiveness. However, this lower rate of antibodies against infliximab has not translated into better effectiveness with methotrexate.

drug in the evening before bed, by taking a supplement of the vitamin folic acid on the day that methotrexate is taken, or by taking an antinausea medication.

Liver Damage
Monitoring of liver blood tests is necessary while a patient takes the drug because methotrexate can result in liver damage and scarring. If the tests are abnormal, the drug has to be stopped or the dose reduced. The risk of liver damage may be increased by moderate to heavy alcohol consumption. The risk seems to increase the longer a patient takes the medication. Monitoring of the blood counts is also required, as it is for azathioprine or 6-MP, but the drug can usually be started at the indicated dose without significant risk.

Allergic Pneumonia
Another side effect that may be rarely experienced in patients receiving methotrexate is allergic pneumonia. If a patient taking methotrexate experiences coughing and shortness of breath, further investigation is usually necessary to look for possible pneumonia.

Cyclosporine

Cyclosporine is a very potent immunosuppressant medication often used in transplant patients to prevent rejection of the transplanted organ. It has been tested in both ulcerative colitis and Crohn's disease. While cyclosporine appears to have no role in the treatment of Crohn's disease, it does bring severe disease flares under control in ulcerative colitis.

Treatment Regimen

Cyclosporine is usually given at first as a continuous intravenous infusion. The intravenous treatment continues until the patient begins to improve significantly or until it is clear that the patient is not improving and surgery is needed to manage the flare.

When a patient improves significantly on intravenous cyclosporine, this drug is switched to a form that is taken by mouth (Neoral). Once the patient is improving and is on oral medications, they are discharged from hospital and Neoral is continued for approximately 3 to 6 months. In most instances, azathioprine is started when the patient is discharged and it is continued after Neoral is stopped, in order to keep the disease in remission.

Cyclosporine Benefits

- Studies have consistently shown that cyclosporine is effective in bringing severe disease flares under reasonable control in ulcerative colitis.

- Cyclosporine is an option for patients who have tried most of the other medical treatments for their disease and found them either unsuccessful or unacceptable because of side effects.

- Cyclosporine is used almost exclusively in hospitalized patients with severe attacks of ulcerative colitis, usually when they have not responded to a course of treatment with intravenous steroids.

- Cyclosporine may "buy" patients some time to get the disease under better control before surgery, even if only temporarily, to get out of hospital, and to think more about the options available to them. In general, people feel better about their decisions, whether it is to go for surgery or to continue trying medical treatment, if they have some time to reflect and if the decisions are not made under duress.

Last Resort

Cyclosporine is not used early in the treatment of ulcerative colitis due to its potential to cause serious side effects. Even with the best medical treatments to maintain remission, approximately 50% of patients who require cyclosporine to bring a severe flare under control end up needing surgery within 1 year.

Side Effects

Cyclosporine should be prescribed only by doctors who are familiar with its use and know how to monitor patients receiving it and what side effects to look for. Serious infections and kidney damage are possible serious side effects. Other side effects from cyclosporine use are high blood pressure, tremor, seizure, and increased hair growth (not usually in places where you want hair to grow).

Serious Infections

As with other immunosuppressant medications, cyclosporine can increase susceptibility to infections. This appears to be more so with cyclosporine than with many of the other immunosuppressant medications.

There are cases of patients developing unusual or rare infections that would not otherwise be seen in someone whose immune system is not being suppressed. Some of these infections can even be fatal, particularly if not detected and treated early. They can occur without a reduction in the white blood cells that help to fight infection. As a result, monitoring the white blood cell count on blood testing cannot predict who will run into this type of complication.

Kidney Damage

When cyclosporine is given, it is usual practice to monitor the levels of the drug in the bloodstream. This is done on a daily basis when the treatment is first started, and although it can be done less frequently once a patient is switched to the capsule form, it must still be continued as long as a patient is receiving the medication. Monitoring the blood levels is important in reducing the risk of kidney damage from the cyclosporine, but it is not a guarantee.

Non-Biologic (Small-Molecule) Drugs

Drugs such as steroids, sulfasalazine, 5-ASA, azathioprine, methotrexate, and cyclosporine are different from the newer types of biologic drugs that have been developed for the treatment of IBD over the past two decades. Unlike the biologics, they are not proteins; they are much smaller in size than the biologic drugs and are typically not broken down and inactivated in the stomach or small intestine, as proteins would be. These drugs are absorbed into the body when taken by mouth, or they act locally on the inner lining of the intestine to reduce inflammation. As a result, they can be taken as pills or capsules and still be effective in treating IBD.

There are some clear potential advantages to non-biologic therapies; the trouble is, the older non-biologic drugs either do not work very well or are associated with a lot of side effects. In recent years, there has been new interest in developing and testing non-biologic drugs that have a more targeted effect on the immune system, resulting in similar effectiveness and safety levels as the biologic drugs, but with the convenience that they can be taken in pill form. One class of these new non-biologic therapies, the Janus kinase inhibitors, is discussed below.

Janus Kinase (JAK) Inhibitors

Janus kinase (JAK) inhibitors are drugs that block the activity of the enzyme JAK, which is involved in the regulation of the body's immune response. Several JAK inhibitor drugs have been developed or are under development for the treatment of various blood disorders and inflammatory conditions, including IBD.

A number of subtypes of the JAK enzyme exist in the body, and different JAK inhibitors may affect the action of these subtypes to a different extent. These variances may have an impact on the effectiveness of a particular drug in treating IBD, and they have also been found to be an important influence on the possible side effects of the drug.

Tofacitinib (Xeljanz) was the first of the JAK inhibitors to be found effective for the treatment of IBD and has been approved for use by regulatory authorities in several countries. It has been shown to be effective in treating ulcerative colitis. It has not been properly tested in Crohn's disease, but some of the other JAK inhibitors, including filgotinib and upadacitinib, are undergoing effectiveness studies for Crohn's disease.

> ### No Antibodies
>
> Because non-biologic drugs consist of comparatively small molecules that are not proteins, the body's immune system does not see them as a potential danger and does not produce antibodies against them. This is a benefit, because antibodies can result in side effects or can cause a biologic drug to stop working.

Tofacitinib Benefits

- In ulcerative colitis, tofacitinib can reduce inflammation and bring a flare under control.
- If tofacitinib is continued after a flare settles, it can decrease the chance of another flare occurring.
- Because the JAK inhibitors are small molecules, and are not proteins, they can be given by mouth in a pill or capsule form.

Side Effects

The JAK inhibitors appear to be relatively well tolerated. They are not steroids, so they do not have all of the potential side effects that are often associated with steroids. However, they do suppress the body's immune response, resulting in an increased risk of infection.

Other side effects seem to depend on which JAK subtype is affected by the drug. In some cases, there is the potential for increased blood lipids, such as cholesterol; in others, there is a possibility of blood count abnormalities or changes in kidney function. These need to be monitored with blood testing.

Shingles

One infection that has been seen more often than expected in people taking tofacitinib is shingles, a painful skin rash triggered by the same virus that causes chicken pox. It is usually localized to one area of the skin, but can be quite painful and can leave a person with pain and skin discoloration even after the infection has cleared. Fortunately, there is a vaccination that reduces the chance of getting shingles, but it isn't yet known whether it is effective in people taking tofacitinib or other JAK inhibitors.

Biologic Drugs

In the late 1990s, infliximab (Remicade), the first biologic drug for the treatment of IBD, was developed and tested. Since then, several more biologic drugs have been found to be effective for IBD. Biologics are quite different from the drugs that preceded them in the treatment of IBD — drugs like steroids, sulfasalazine, 5-ASA, azathioprine, and methotrexate. The biologic drugs are designed either to block specific molecules or receptors on cells that are important in promoting intestinal inflammation, or to activate other molecules or receptors that are key players in reducing intestinal inflammation. They have the potential to provide very targeted treatment.

The biologic drugs are proteins, or parts of a protein, and are much larger and more complex than the previously available drugs. As a result, they are more difficult to develop and to manufacture. Their development and production require special technology known as genetic engineering, so they are sometimes called designer drugs. They are engineered to specifically target key parts of the immune response that promote inflammation in IBD while potentially leaving other parts of the immune response unaffected. The older types of

---

First Biologic Therapy

Infliximab was the first biologic therapy approved for use in IBD, and it is very effective at treating several forms of IBD. It was approved for use in Crohn's disease in 1998 in the United States and in 2001 in Canada. It was approved for ulcerative colitis in both countries a few years later.

---

medication are thought to be much less selective in what they target. Theoretically, therefore, biologic drugs may be more effective and could have fewer side effects.

Because of the large size of the molecules that make up biologic drugs, and because they are proteins, getting them into the bloodstream and the body tissues can also be a challenge. They cannot be absorbed into the body if they are taken by mouth in a pill or capsule form. In addition, if they are taken by mouth, the protein will be broken down and inactivated by the acid in the stomach and by the digestive processes of the small intestine. Thus, biologic drugs must be given as an intravenous infusion directly into a vein or as an injection using a needle under the skin. This may be a disadvantage for people who find injections or intravenous treatments to be painful or inconvenient.

Another potential drawback is that, because a biologic drug is a large protein and because it is not normally produced in the human body, a person's immune system may see it as being "foreign" or a potential danger and may develop antibodies against it. This is how the immune system protects us against infections — by producing antibodies against the proteins on viruses and bacteria; the antibodies help to remove or kill the viruses or bacteria. However, when antibodies develop against a biologic drug, they can attach to the drug and prevent it from working or cause it to be removed from the body more quickly, which can reduce or prevent the drug's effectiveness in treating IBD.

Tumor Necrosis Factor Alpha (TNF-Alpha) Blockers

The first type of biologic drugs developed for the treatment of IBD were designed to inactivate or block the effects of a protein called tumor necrosis factor alpha (TNF-alpha). They are often called TNF inhibitors or anti-TNF therapies. They are highly effective at treating several forms of IBD.

Although they are very similar in how they work, there are some potentially important differences among the various TNF-alpha blockers that may make a particular one the preferred choice in a certain situation.

Infliximab (Remicade, Inflectra, Remsima)

Infliximab is an antibody, produced using genetic technology, composed of part human protein and part mouse protein. It attaches to and inactivates a protein called tumor necrosis factor alpha (TNF-alpha). TNF-alpha is a critically important protein in the process of causing inflammation. Blocking its action results in improvement in intestinal inflammation and improved symptoms of IBD.

Treatment Regimen

Because the infliximab antibody is itself a protein, it cannot be taken by mouth. Rather, it is given as intravenous infusions, usually over a period of 1 to 2 hours, in an infusion clinic or other outpatient facility.

The initial course of treatment prescribed may vary from physician to physician. Some prescribe one or possibly two infusions given 2 to 4 weeks apart and then assess the response to treatment before deciding on the usefulness of further treatments. Others give a "standard" three-dose "induction regimen" involving an initial infusion, a second one 2 weeks later, and a third one 4 weeks after the second. Following the third infusion, the response is assessed and further treatment decisions made.

Patients who are very sick and are hospitalized because of their IBD may be treated with higher-than-standard doses of infliximab, given more frequently than usual.

Once an IBD sufferer has responded to an initial course of infliximab, repeated dosing with infliximab — usually every 6 to 8 weeks — will help maintain the initial improvement. Doctors will often order a blood test that measures the amount of infliximab in the bloodstream just before a dose is given. The drug level will often provide some guidance about how frequently infliximab should be administered and whether the dose needs to be increased or, in the occasional case, decreased.

We know from clinical trials that infliximab continues to reduce the risk of relapse or flare for at least 1 year after treatment is first started. Although there is really no information from the clinical studies about what happens after 1 year, it has been the experience of many doctors treating patients with infliximab that flares tend to occur more often if the treatment is stopped even after 1 year.

The response to infliximab can be very impressive, and it may seem that the disease has been "cured," but once infliximab is stopped, the risk of recurrent symptoms goes up. There does not appear to be a clear "exit strategy" for the majority of patients when infliximab treatment is started. This may be difficult for both patients and doctors to accept, but the facts that Crohn's disease and ulcerative colitis are chronic disorders and that infliximab is a treatment and not a cure must be kept in mind. It works only as long as it is taken.

Dosing Effect

Repeated dosing of infliximab can produce complete healing of the inner lining of the intestine, something that is not consistently observed with any of the previous medical therapies, with the possible exception of azathioprine and 6-MP. It also appears that the use of infliximab can result in a reduction in the need for hospitalization and surgery for individuals with Crohn's disease.

Naveen returns to see his gastro-enterologist 2 weeks later to review the test results. He is feeling better since starting prednisone, with less diarrhea and abdominal cramping, but he is still seeing blood in the stool and feeling tired.

The doctor tells Naveen that the MRI confirmed the ultrasound results but it also showed that he has two separate segments of small intestine that are inflamed. One is about 20 inches (50 cm) long, in the last part of the small intestine (the terminal ileum); the other is a bit farther up the small intestine and is about 12 inches (30 cm) long. She tells him this means he has extensive disease and should really go on a biologic drug and not wait to see how he fares on prednisone.

She recommends a TNF-alpha blocker, such as infliximab or adalimumab, because she has confidence that these drugs can potentially reverse some of the areas of inflammation seen in the colonoscopy and MRI enterography, and thereby reduce the chance that he will need surgery in the future. She recognizes that, if he ends up needing surgery, it will be very complicated and extensive, and may leave him with problems absorbing fluids and nutrients from his diet, or could leave him with an ostomy.

Naveen is concerned about going on such a strong drug and about possible side effects, since his doctor has told him he will likely need to stay on the drug for several years. He is particularly worried because doctors have not had as much experience with TNF-alpha blockers as they have with drugs like prednisone. But his doctor explains that the risk of a serious side effect is very small — about 1 chance in 5,000 — whereas the risk that he will require surgery if his Crohn's disease is not properly controlled with medication is likely greater than 50%. With the situation described that way, Naveen chooses to go ahead with a TNF-alpha blocker.

Antibodies

Some patients receiving infliximab will develop antibodies directed against it after receiving several doses. These are often called antidrug antibodies. Antibodies may increase the risk of certain side effects and, in some cases where antibodies form, there is a decrease in the length of time of the perceived beneficial effect. Initially, the beneficial effect of an infusion may last for 8 weeks before symptoms start to recur, but when antibodies to infliximab develop, this may drop down to 6 weeks or even 4 weeks.

In some instances, infliximab appears to stop working altogether. In those cases, using another TNF-alpha blocker that is entirely human protein — and presumably would not be blocked by antibodies against infliximab — may be effective at regaining a beneficial effect. Currently, adalimumab (Humira)

Foreign Protein

Because infliximab is "foreign" protein (partly human and partly mouse protein), this may activate the immune system to produce antibodies directed against infliximab. These antibodies can result in an increase in infusion reactions, and may also result in a loss of the effectiveness of infliximab over time.

is the only completely human TNF-alpha blocker that is approved for use in both Crohn's disease and ulcerative colitis in the United States and Canada. Golimumab (Simponi), another human TNF-alpha blocker, is approved for use only in ulcerative colitis, although many doctors have found that it is also effective in Crohn's disease.

Infliximab Benefits

- In clinical trials, infliximab was first found to be effective in treating symptoms of active Crohn's disease: 60% to 80% of patients responded positively. Improvement appears to occur very quickly in many patients, often within days of a single dose, with patients sometimes experiencing an improvement in their overall sense of well-being, energy, and appetite within hours of a dose.

- Many of the patients who were first studied in the clinical trials were on other medications for their Crohn's disease — 5-ASA drugs, steroids, or immunosuppressants — and had not noticed a significant response to these treatments until they were given infliximab. These patients, sometimes described by physicians as "treatment resistant," pose the greatest challenge to doctors treating Crohn's disease. These are the patients who most frequently require hospitalization and surgery.

- Infliximab has also been found to be effective in the treatment of fistulas due to Crohn's disease. Previously, there was no proven effective treatment for this troubling complication, although antibiotics can often reduce some of the pain and drainage over the short term. Infliximab is the first treatment shown to cause fistulas to stop draining, and, with repeated dosing, infliximab can prevent drainage from recurring. Whether the fistulas treated with infliximab actually heal (that is, the channel actually closes up) or just stop draining, with the channel remaining present and open, is a matter of considerable controversy. However, from a patient's perspective, the distinction is not pressing since the important outcome is the elimination of pain and drainage from the fistula.

- Two large studies have shown that infliximab is effective in treating patients with active ulcerative colitis who have not responded to other ulcerative colitis treatments — once again, the "treatment resistant" patients. It appears that repeated dosing every 8 weeks helps maintain the initial improvement that is seen with infliximab in about 60% of patients.

- Infliximab has become the treatment of choice for patients who are hospitalized with a severe flare of ulcerative colitis and who are not responding to several days of intravenous steroids. These patients are facing a very high likelihood of needing surgery if infliximab is not used; even with infliximab, many of them do not respond well enough to avoid surgery. Research is ongoing on how to provide the optimal dosing of infliximab to these very sick patients.

The same blood test that measures the infliximab level in the bloodstream can also test for antibodies. In most cases where there are antibodies against infliximab, the amount of infliximab in the bloodstream is much too low; in some cases, it is undetectable.

Short-Term Safety

Since its release, infliximab has been used extensively throughout the world, not just in IBD but also in rheumatoid arthritis and a number of other disorders. The short-term safety record has been excellent. This is not to say that there aren't potential side effects, but these tend to be relatively rare events or relatively mild and easily manageable.

Infusion Reaction

The most common side effect is an acute reaction that occurs in 5% to 10% of patients during the infusion process, most commonly experienced as flushing, warmth, and redness along with a feeling of chest tightness and shortness of breath. This does not appear to be an allergic reaction, but may be related to how quickly the medication is infused.

Although the reaction may be quite distressing, it is never serious or life-threatening. This reaction always goes away after stopping the infusion temporarily and administering an antihistamine or acetaminophen (Tylenol). Once the reaction has been settled, the infusion can be resumed at a slower rate. As the infusion progresses, the speed of the infusion can usually be increased again. These reactions can be prevented by antihistamine or steroid medication taken just prior to the infliximab infusion.

Infections

Infliximab may affect the immune system in a way that makes a person more susceptible to certain infections, most notably tuberculosis. Soon after infliximab was approved for use in Crohn's disease and rheumatoid arthritis, a number of cases of tuberculosis were noted in patients receiving this treatment. Many of these cases occurred within 3 months of starting infliximab. Once this was recognized, patients embarking on infliximab treatment have commonly been tested for tuberculosis by means of a skin test and possibly a chest X-ray. If tuberculosis is detected, treatment of the tuberculosis is generally recommended prior to starting infliximab. This has resulted in a significant reduction in the rate of tuberculosis, back down to the rate that was observed before infliximab was introduced on the market.

> **Due Caution**
>
> There may still be other unusual infections that can occur in patients receiving infliximab and that cannot be screened for by means of skin tests or chest X-rays. Every patient receiving infliximab should report to a doctor any unusual symptoms, such as a cough or severe and persistent headache, especially if they are associated with a fever.

Q What drugs are safe for women who have IBD and become pregnant?

A None of the drugs that are used for IBD is known without a doubt to be safe in pregnancy because the types of studies needed to prove complete safety have not been done and are unlikely to ever be done. Despite this, there is a considerable amount of experience using most of the drugs, and there does not appear to be any evidence of increased risk to the pregnancy or to the fetus with most drugs used for IBD. The one definite exception is methotrexate, which has been definitively shown to cause spontaneous abortions and malformations of the fetus.

Because they have been available as IBD treatments for a much shorter time, there is less experience with the use of the biologic drugs and the newer small-molecule drugs, such as tofacitinib, in pregnancy. However, in the time that the TNF-alpha blockers infliximab and adalimumab have been on the market, a substantial number of women have been treated with these drugs, and there does not appear to be any increased risk of bad pregnancy outcomes or congenital malformations. These drugs do pass from the mother's bloodstream into the fetus in the last trimester of pregnancy, and can be found in the baby's bloodstream even 9 months after delivery in some cases. So far, this has not resulted in any reported side effects for the infants of mothers receiving a TNF-alpha blocker. However, it is generally recommended that infants do not receive live vaccines during the first 6 to 9 months of life if their mothers were taking these drugs in the last trimester of pregnancy, because a baby's immune system could potentially be suppressed and it is theoretically possible that a live vaccine could actually cause an infection. The transfer of drug from mother to baby has raised questions regarding whether infliximab, adalimumab, and golimumab should be temporarily stopped during the final months of pregnancy.

There is considerable controversy surrounding this issue and, although it appears that the drug might be able to be stopped for a few months at the end of pregnancy without a huge risk of IBD flare, the risk does seem to increase the longer the woman is off treatment. In addition, if antitumor necrosis factor therapy is restarted after a gap of several months, there may be an increased risk of subsequent allergic reactions and possibly reduced long-term effectiveness of the drug. These factors need to be considered by the woman and her doctor when deciding on what to do about therapy with TNF-alpha blockers in the later stages of pregnancy.

The other antitumor necrosis factor alpha drug, certolizumab pegol (Cimzia), does not appear to cross over to the baby's circulation during pregnancy and may provide some theoretical advantage over the other two drugs during pregnancy. However, in most instances where a pregnant woman is already taking infliximab or adalimumab during pregnancy and doing well from the perspective of her IBD, it is not advisable to switch medications.

Long-Term Safety

Although most physicians caring for IBD patients in any significant numbers feel comfortable with the short-term safety record and the potential benefits of infliximab and other commonly used TNF-alpha blockers, such as adalimumab (Humira) and golimumab (Simponi), there are still some reservations about the possibility of long-term effects that will become apparent only after many years of use.

Infliximab was first used in clinical trials in the mid-1990s, and as a result there is some reasonable long-term follow-up on many patients to provide us with some early long-term safety information. At this time, there is no conclusive evidence that infliximab produces an increase in late effects, such as cancer. Nevertheless, in the United States, infliximab has been given a label that indicates an association with an increased risk of lymphoma, a relatively rare form of cancer of the lymph glands. Although there is no direct proof that infliximab carries this risk, there is evidence that other drugs designed to block the action of TNF-alpha may increase the risk of lymphoma in patients with rheumatoid arthritis. To some extent, this is akin to "guilt by association." The complete story will take several years to unfold, but there is currently no reason to avoid the use of infliximab due to a theoretical risk of lymphoma.

While there is no solid direct proof that infliximab by itself causes lymphoma, a particularly rare form of lymphoma that occurs primarily in young males has been linked to the use of TNF-alpha blockers. However, this type of lymphoma has been seen only in patients who took immune-suppressive drugs, such as azathioprine or 6-mercaptopurine, in combination with a TNF-alpha blocker. In the absence of immune-suppressive drugs, this type of lymphoma is not seen in patients receiving TNF-alpha blockers. Because this type of lymphoma is particularly aggressive and catastrophic, many doctors avoid using azathioprine or 6-mercaptopurine with TNF-alpha blockers even though there is evidence that the combination may enhance the effectiveness of the TNF-alpha blocker.

Adalimumab (Humira)

Adalimumab is an antibody against TNF-alpha that, unlike infliximab, which contains some mouse protein, is an entirely human antibody. When given to an individual, the adalimumab antibody is still seen by the immune system as being "foreign" and, as a result, can still cause formation of antibodies against the drug. However, the formation of antibodies against the drug appears to be less frequent with adalimumab than with infliximab. Like infliximab, adalimumab is effective in the

Convenience

Unlike infliximab, which is given by an intravenous infusion, adalimumab is given by an injection under the skin every 1 to 2 weeks. As a result, it offers some advantages in terms of convenience for patients who can be taught to do the injections themselves rather than having to go to a clinic or hospital where the infusion of infliximab is given.

short- and long-term treatment of Crohn's disease and in some patients with ulcerative colitis.

Because adalimumab is not given by an intravenous infusion, it does not carry the risk of an infusion reaction as does infliximab. However, there is sometimes some local pain and redness at the site of adalimumab injection. This occurs only in a small minority of patients and is usually mild and not long-lasting.

Golimumab (Simponi)

Golimumab is another antibody that has been developed against TNF-alpha. Like adalimumab, it is entirely human. Although antibodies can develop against golimumab, it happens very infrequently. Golimumab is administered as an injection under the skin, usually twice in 2 weeks and then once every 4 weeks. It is effective for the treatment of flares of ulcerative colitis, and for those people who experience improvement on golimumab, continuing its use helps to maintain the improvement.

Golimumab has not been approved for the treatment of Crohn's disease, but that is because there have been no clinical trials designed and carried out to determine if it is an effective and safe treatment for Crohn's disease. Nevertheless, some physicians have prescribed golimumab for their Crohn's disease patients, with some good results.

Certolizumab Pegol (Cimzia)

Certolizumab pegol is a biologic therapy that was developed to block the action of TNF-alpha, similar to infliximab, adalimumab, and golimumab. It is different from these three drugs in that it is not a complete antibody but is only a fragment of an antibody that is attached to a large molecule called PEG in order to slow down its elimination from the body. As with adalimumab and golimumab, it is given by subcutaneous injection, initially three times over a 4-week period, and then once every 4 weeks. It has been shown to be effective in Crohn's disease treatment but has been approved for use for this indication only in the United States and Switzerland.

Other Biologic Therapies

Vedolizumab (Entyvio)

Vedolizumab is a biologic drug that, unlike the other biologic drugs that are used to treat IBD, was developed to treat only IBD; it is not used to treat other inflammatory conditions, such as arthritis. The reason it is used to treat only IBD is that it is "gut specific" by virtue of the fact that it consists of an

---

No Infusion Reactions

Like infliximab or adalimumab, golimumab increases the risk of infections; however, because it is not given by intravenous infusion, the infusion reactions seen with infliximab do not occur with golimumab.

antibody that attaches to white blood cells in the bloodstream and prevents them from getting from the bloodstream into the intestine, where they cause inflammation. What makes vedolizumab so unique is the fact that it does not prevent the white blood cells from getting into other tissues in the body; as a result, it does not appear to suppress the entire body's immune system, only the immune system of the gut.

The overall result is that it reduces inflammation in the intestine of patients with Crohn's disease and ulcerative colitis, but does not result in an increased risk of infection or other side effects usually associated with the use of immune-suppressant medications. This theoretical advantage of vedolizumab has been borne out in day-to-day use, with serious infections occurring only very rarely. When they do occur, it is difficult to make a connection between vedolizumab treatment and the infection.

Vedolizumab is given by intravenous infusion, usually every 8 weeks, but occasionally as often as every 4 weeks.

> ### The Unknowns
>
> It is not known whether vedolizumab is effective against some of the complications of IBD that occur outside of the intestine — things like arthritis, skin reactions, and liver complications — or if it has any effect on the fistula complications that can occur with Crohn's disease.

Vedolizumab Benefits

- Vedolizumab is effective at treating the symptoms of a flare of ulcerative colitis or Crohn's disease.
- If it is continued beyond the initial treatment period of 6 weeks, vedolizumab can result in further reduction of symptoms and can help reduce the chance that symptoms of a flare will return.
- Vedolizumab suppresses the immune system of the gut, but not that of the entire body.

Ustekinumab (Stelara)

Ustekinumab is another biologic drug that has been proven to be an effective treatment for Crohn's disease, but so far it has not been adequately tested in ulcerative colitis. It is an antibody that attaches to and blocks the action of two proteins, called interleukin-12 and interleukin-23. These proteins produce increased inflammation in tissues; when their action is blocked by ustekinumab, inflammation caused by Crohn's disease is reduced.

Ustekinumab has not been tested in ulcerative colitis, but in Crohn's disease, it brings symptoms of a flare under control. The first treatment is typically given as an intravenous infusion. After the first intravenous dose, ustekinumab is usually given as an injection under the skin every 8 weeks. This injection can be administered by the patient or by a family member.

Psoriasis

Well before it was shown to be effective for treating Crohn's disease, ustekinumab was known to be a very good treatment for psoriasis, an inflammatory condition of the skin that results in itchy and unsightly scaly rashes.

Ustekinumab has very few noticeable side effects that would bother someone taking it. However, it does suppress the body's immune response to some degree; as a result, there is a small increase in the risk of infections. This increased risk is likely not much different from the risk that goes along with many of the other immune-suppressant drugs used to treat IBD.

Ustekinumab Benefits

- In Crohn's disease, ustekinumab helps control the symptoms of a flare.
- If ustekinumab is continued after the first treatment, it can help maintain the improvement in symptoms.
- For people who were taking steroid therapy for Crohn's disease without significant improvement, ustekinumab can help them reduce their dose of steroids or get off them completely.

Other Interleukin-12 and Interleukin-23 Inhibitors

There are a number of other drugs that block the action of both interleukin-12 and interleukin-23, or just the action of interleukin-23. These drugs are under development and are being tested for use in IBD and other diseases, and there are early indications that some of them may be effective. Only further testing and clinical trials will determine their place in the treatment of Crohn's disease and ulcerative colitis.

Biosimilars

When the patent expires on a brand-name drug, other companies will copy the drug to manufacture and sell it. These copies are called generic drugs, and they are usually much less expensive than the brand-name drug, in part because the companies that make them don't have to carry out the rigorous, very costly, and time-consuming testing that is required to get a new medication approved for the treatment of a given condition or illness. Rather, they need only show that their drug is chemically identical to the brand-name drug and is identical in the way it is handled by the body.

Generic drugs have been used to treat everything from high blood pressure and high cholesterol to heart disease and inflammatory bowel disease. However, producing an exact copy of a drug is really only feasible for the small-molecule drugs. The biologic drugs are much larger molecules and are much more complex. Although biologics can't be copied to produce a true generic drug, highly similar drugs that replicate many or most aspects of a specific biologic drug can be produced. These are often called biosimilars.

The regulations regarding the approval of biosimilar drugs vary somewhat from country to country. In general, a biosimilar must be proven to be highly similar to the original biologic drug (often called the originator) with respect to its chemical structure and what it does in experimental model systems that test important biological properties of the drug. In most countries, the biosimilar drug must undergo clinical trial testing comparing it to the originator in a human disease or condition for which the originator is approved for use. If the biosimilar is shown to be highly similar — that is, there are no important differences when it is used to treat a human disease — it can then be approved for use in that disease.

In most cases, the biosimilar is then also approved for use in all of the other conditions for which the originator is approved. An example is the development of an infliximab biosimilar that was first tested in the lab and found to be almost chemically indistinguishable from the infliximab originator (Remicade).

More to Come

Remicade is the first biologic drug for the treatment of IBD for which there is a biosimilar (called Inflectra or Remsima), but there are certainly more to come as other biologic drugs lose their patent protection.

The Cost Factor

Biosimilars have the potential to help limit the rapidly increasing cost of drug treatment for IBD, as they are generally substantially less costly than the originator biologic drugs. However, the issue of biosimilars brings out a lot of strong feelings among people with IBD and their families, particularly those who are already on an originator biologic, such as Remicade, and doing well. They are concerned that the insurance plan that is paying for their medications will force them to switch from the originator to the biosimilar. This may be perfectly safe to do without a significant risk of an IBD flare, but an individual may be unwilling to take even an extremely small risk. They may ask, "Why should I switch my medication when I am doing so well? Just so my insurance plan can save some money?" In some ways, they are correct. However, there may be cost benefits to the individual, too, particularly if they are paying out of pocket for a portion of their medication or if their insurance plan has a lifetime cap on the amount that can be spent on drugs.

The effectiveness and safety of the biosimilar infliximab was then compared with those of Remicade in people with rheumatoid arthritis, a condition for which infliximab is approved. The results were almost indistinguishable between the two drugs, and biosimilar infliximab received regulatory approval in many countries for all of the conditions for which Remicade is used. This approval included Crohn's disease and ulcerative colitis, even though the biosimilar infliximab had not been tested in IBD. Since then, it has become apparent that biosimilar infliximab is not different from Remicade in any important way when used in Crohn's disease and ulcerative colitis.

Future Medical Therapies

The causes of abnormal inflammation and damage in the intestine of an individual with ulcerative colitis or Crohn's disease are very complicated, and there are many steps in the normal control of inflammation and the repair of damaged tissues during which problems can occur. New treatments that aim to correct those problems are likely to be developed over the coming years and may become available for the treatment of IBD. Some of these developments will almost certainly be guided by what we learn from studies of the underlying causes of IBD.

Treatments That Target the Microbiome

There is a lot of evidence that bacteria in the intestine are, in some way, related to the development of IBD. Experiments in animal models of IBD have clearly shown that bacteria are necessary for colitis to occur. In humans, the types and variety of bacteria that are present in the intestines of people with IBD are different from those found in people who don't have IBD. There are particular bacterial species or strains that seem to protect against inflammation and others that seem to cause or increase inflammation.

It is clear that the bacterial community in the intestine — the so-called gut microbiome — is somehow involved in the development of IBD. As a result of these observations, there has been considerable interest in developing therapies for IBD that somehow alter the gut microbiome.

Probiotics
Probiotics are bacteria that are thought to have health-maintaining or health-promoting properties. They are available in numerous commercially available products that contain millions or billions of bacteria. Some contain a single

bacterial species or strain, while others contain a combination of different strains, to try to maximize the potential health benefits. The bacteria in probiotics are supposed to be live, or at least be in a dormant state with the ability to become active once in a person's intestine.

Several probiotics have been tested in IBD, with somewhat inconsistent results. A bacterial strain called E. coli Nissle has been tested in patients with ulcerative colitis whose disease was in remission, and was found to be about as effective at reducing the chance of a flare as taking a 5-ASA medication.

Another probiotic that is popular among IBD patients is VSL#3, a combination of eight different bacterial strains put together into a powder that is taken by mouth. It has been studied primarily in people with ulcerative colitis who have had their colon surgically removed and a "pelvic pouch" created using a portion of the remaining small intestine. These patients sometimes develop inflammation in the pouch, with symptoms that are very much like the symptoms of ulcerative colitis. VSL#3 has been found, in some studies, to prevent the development of pouchitis — inflammation of the pouch — and to reduce symptoms in people who have pouchitis.

Aside from the E. coli Nissle probiotic, there is no evidence that any probiotic, including VSL#3, is effective in improving outcomes in ulcerative colitis or Crohn's disease. For many people with pouchitis who take VSL#3, their experience is not as positive as the results that have been reported in some clinical trials. Furthermore, when taken in the doses studied in the clinical trials, probiotic treatment can be relatively expensive, and it is not covered by drug insurance plans.

Despite the fact that there is limited hard evidence to support the use of probiotics in treating IBD, they do appear to be extremely safe and certainly address a possible mechanism of disease that traditional drug therapies do not. This appeals to many IBD sufferers and merits further study.

Fecal Microbial Transplantation

A form of bacterial therapy that has gained a lot of attention is fecal microbial transplantation (FMT). The idea behind it is similar to that of probiotic therapy, but instead of the patient ingesting a limited number of bacterial strains packed into a capsule or powder, FMT takes all of the different bacterial strains present in the large intestine of a healthy person (the donor) and transplants them into someone suffering from ulcerative colitis or Crohn's disease (the recipient). The goal is to reestablish a more "normal" microbiome in the IBD patient and control the inflammation and symptoms. The hope is that

> **Burden of Evidence**
>
> Because probiotics are not considered medications, the manufacturers of probiotics are not necessarily required to provide the same amount or the same quality of evidence that pharmaceutical companies must provide in order to prove the effectiveness and safety of their drugs before they come to market.

the normalization of the microbiome and the improvement in IBD will both be long-lasting.

The problem is that there is huge variation in how FMT is carried out; as a result, it becomes very difficult to interpret the results of studies that have tried to determine whether FMT is an effective and safe treatment for IBD. Major areas of variation include who the donor is, how their stool sample is processed, and how and when it is administered to the recipient. These factors — especially who the donor is — have been shown to significantly affect the results obtained with FMT.

Some studies have administered the transplant by injecting the solution containing the bacteria into the colon through a colonoscope; others have given it by enema; still others have delivered it via a tube run through the nose down into the stomach and the small intestine. In addition, different studies have administered the FMT at different time points — varying the amount of time that elapses between when the stool sample is taken from the donor and when the transplant is given to the recipient — and at different frequencies, making interpretation and comparison of results even more difficult.

A potential concern with FMT is its safety. Since billions of bacteria are transplanted from the donor into the recipient, it is possible that some of them could cause disease. Another worrisome possibility is that other microbes, such as viruses, could also be transmitted. Some of the viruses of concern are HIV and hepatitis. Donors are usually screened for these types of viruses and infections, but screening is not always 100% accurate and there is a potential risk (though likely quite small) of the transplantation of a disease-causing bacteria or virus that is not being screened for. One way that doctors performing FMT have minimized this risk is by using a close family member of the recipient as the donor. Patients are usually more comfortable getting the transplant from a family member than from a complete stranger.

So far, despite all of the interest and theory behind it, FMT is far from proven as an effective and safe therapy for IBD. It is quite possible that it will be found to be effective in some situations and for some forms of IBD, but many of the details still need to be worked out.

Freeze-Dried Preparations

Freeze-dried FMT preparations have been developed, allowing for live bacteria to be stored for longer periods before they are administered. Without freeze-drying, the transplant must be carried out within a few hours of obtaining the stool sample from the donor, which makes FMT difficult to coordinate from a practical standpoint.

Complementary and Alternative Medicine

Although there have been important advances in the treatment of Crohn's disease and ulcerative colitis with the development of new and effective medications, there are still some people with IBD who do not have good control of their disease with drug therapy and continue to have symptoms despite treatment. These people will sometimes turn to other, non-traditional ways to manage their condition or their symptoms.

Nontraditional therapies are known as complementary and alternative medicine, or CAM. This term encompasses a wide range of different forms of therapy, from marijuana to massage. Depending on how CAM is defined, studies have shown that up to half of IBD sufferers have tried CAM at some point in the course of their disease. Some people choose to try a form of CAM not because they have exhausted all forms of traditional drug therapy but because they have concerns about the impact drug therapy will have on their body or their immune system, or because CAM fits better with their own view of their disease and they perceive it as being safer or more "natural."

Many of the therapies used as part of CAM consist of plant-based products or extracts. It is certainly possible that these therapies could have some effect on IBD. Some of the medications that have been used in traditional Western medicine are derived from plants, so it does not take a huge leap to believe that some plant-derived products might be anti-inflammatory or might help protect the intestinal lining and, as a result, provide some benefit to people suffering with IBD. Many IBD sufferers report an improvement in symptoms when they try natural products; some even claim they are able to remain in good health and off all medication while taking them. Unfortunately, there is very little evidence to support these observations and claims, and very few types of CAM have been tested in a scientific way that would enable us to conclude whether they are effective and safe to use in IBD.

One of the problems with CAM is that many doctors are not familiar with it because it is not given much emphasis in the curriculum of most medical schools or specialty training programs, and because no scientifically sound studies have been carried out to properly assess the numerous possible therapies. As a result, many doctors feel that they are unable to make a recommendation for the use of CAM to manage IBD.

Safety of CAM

Many people consider CAM to be safer or more natural than traditional drug therapy, but that is not necessarily the case. Just because something is "natural," or plant-based, does not mean it is safe. Many natural health products are not subjected to the same safety testing and quality control that are required of traditional drugs. However, most of the natural products that are commonly tried by IBD patients appear to be quite safe, although side effects have sometimes been reported.

Rebecca is a 34-year-old woman who is the manager of a natural health products store. After experiencing pains in the right lower part of her abdomen, along with some bloating and nausea, she has been recently diagnosed with Crohn's disease, with involvement of the last part of the small intestine (the terminal ileum).

She had not really experienced much change in her bowel habits or blood in her stool, and her pain was initially suspected to be due to ovarian cysts. However, an ultrasound revealed a thickened segment of small intestine measuring about 6 inches (15 cm) in length. A blood test revealed mild anemia but no iron deficiency, and she has a raised level of C-reactive protein (a marker of inflammation) in her blood.

Rebecca is referred to a gastroenterologist, who suggests a course of budesonide therapy. She reluctantly agrees to it, but it does not seem to have any impact on her symptoms. At her follow-up visit, the gastroenterologist suggests a course of prednisone. Rebecca knows enough about the possible side effects to know that she really does not want to take it. She leaves the appointment without a prescription and without a clear plan of what she is going to do.

She knows that several of the clients of her store have Crohn's disease or ulcerative colitis, and she talks to them about what they have found to be helpful in managing their disease without conventional drug therapy. She gets somewhat different feedback from each of them, but tries a combination of three different naturopathic preparations, none of which seems to affect how often she experiences the pain or how severe the pain is. Rebecca decides to try marijuana as a way to manage her symptoms. She finds that smoking marijuana helps to eliminate her nausea and takes the edge off the pain.

She goes back to see her family doctor, who repeats the blood tests and finds that her C-reactive protein level is still high. The doctor arranges for another ultrasound, and the abnormal segment of small intestine looks virtually the same as it did when Rebecca was first diagnosed with Crohn's disease.

Many patients then turn to CAM practitioners, who may make recommendations that are not based on accepted scientific evidence; nevertheless, these suggestions are often willingly accepted by patients. This is not necessarily a problem, but some patients who choose to try CAM will stop their traditional IBD treatment, perhaps because the traditional therapy is not having the desired effect on their IBD or is causing troublesome side effects; it is more worrisome when a patient stops treatments that are having a beneficial impact on their IBD because they want to give CAM a try.

Marijuana (Cannabis) and the Cannabinoids

It is likely that all doctors who treat people with IBD have had a patient report that smoking, inhaling, or ingesting marijuana helps their IBD. This observation has stimulated interest in the use of cannabinoids — the family of chemicals that produce the effects of marijuana on the nervous system — for the treatment of IBD. A clinical trial found that marijuana helped the symptoms of Crohn's disease, but it did not find that marijuana had any effect on intestinal inflammation. A logical conclusion, when one carefully examines the results, is that marijuana may help with some of the symptoms commonly seen in Crohn's disease, such as loss of appetite, nausea, and abdominal cramping, but it does so through its effect on the brain and possibly also on the nerves connecting to the intestine, not by reducing inflammation or healing the intestine.

Complementary and Alternative Medicine

The following are some of the alternative therapies that are sometimes used by patients for the management of IBD and its symptoms.

Plant-derived therapies

- Aloe vera
- Bilberry
- Boswellia (*Boswellia serrata*)
- Chiretta (*Andrographis paniculata*)
- Curcumin (turmeric)
- Evening primrose oil (*Oenothera biennis*)
- Marijuana (cannabis) and cannabinoids
- Slippery elm bark (*Ulmus rubra*)
- Thunder god vine (*Tripterygium wilfordii*)
- Wheat grass (*Triticum aestivum*)
- Wormwood (absinthe)

Mind-body therapies

- Cognitive therapy
- Guided imagery
- Hypnotherapy
- Mind-body training
- Mindfulness
- Relaxation techniques
- Stress management

Acupuncture and moxibustion

Exercise-based therapies

Massage therapy

Some people consider fecal microbial transplantation, probiotic therapies, and dietary therapies, such as fish oil supplementation, to be forms of CAM. These are discussed in other sections of this book.

A subsequent study, using a cannabinoid derivative of marijuana that does not have an effect on the brain, found no significant impact on Crohn's disease symptoms. At the present time, marijuana can be considered a treatment only for some IBD-related symptoms; there is no evidence that it has any positive effect on the underlying disease.

Mind-Body Therapies

Mind-body therapies include mindfulness, hypnotherapy, cognitive therapy, stress management, relaxation techniques, guided imagery, and mind-body training. In general, these therapies seem to improve depression, anxiety, and psychological well-being, but studies have not consistently found them to have an effect on intestinal inflammation, bowel symptoms, or pain. Nevertheless, many people with IBD find that these therapies help them deal with their disease, its symptoms, and its impact on their psychological well-being.

Clinical Research Study Designs

There are a variety of different clinical study designs, but the most commonly used one is the randomized controlled trial. In this type of study, patients with a given condition (for example, Crohn's disease) are randomly assigned (such as by the flip of a coin) to receive either the "standard therapy" or the "experimental therapy." The patients are then closely watched for a period of time and the outcomes of interest are measured or monitored. An outcome may be, for example, elimination of all symptoms of Crohn's disease. By comparing the proportion of individuals receiving standard therapy and the proportion of individuals receiving experimental therapy who experience elimination of their symptoms, research scientists can make a conclusion about which one works better.

Risk

By definition, you are being experimented upon in this type of trial, but safeguards are put in place to protect your safety. Nevertheless, there is always some inherent risk in participating. This risk should be fully described to you in a patient information and informed consent document, which you will sign before the study begins. This document describes what the study is; who is carrying it out; why it is being carried out; what is involved in participating (for example, number and types of visits, procedures, and tests); what the potential risks are to you in participating; what the potential benefits are to you; what your rights are within the study; and what your rights are should you choose not to participate.

After reading the document, which can often be quite lengthy, you will have the opportunity to ask questions of the study coordinator or the study investigator. If you need to, you can take the document home so that you can look it over again and, if necessary, discuss the study with your family and friends or with another doctor. Before agreeing to participate in a study, you should be comfortable with the decision.

Obligation

You should not feel obliged to participate in the study, and a decision not to participate should not affect the health care that you receive from your doctor. Similarly, if you decide at any point during the course of a clinical study that you no longer wish to participate, your care will not be affected.

New Types of Study Designs

Traditionally, clinical trials have compared one drug against another drug or against a placebo. Newer trial designs have moved toward comparing treatment strategies that may incorporate not only different medications but also the use of laboratory testing to guide therapy. In these studies, medical clinics or practices, rather than individual patients, may be randomly assigned to one of two or more different strategies.

 I have been approached by my doctor to participate in a research study. What's involved in participating in a study? Should I do it? If I do participate, will I be a "guinea pig"? If I don't do it, will my doctor be upset with me?

 Clinical research in IBD is a critically important type of research that is aimed at finding and developing new and better treatments for IBD. It can also help to determine which treatment, among a variety of existing or available treatments, is the best treatment in a given situation. Clinical research is also needed by pharmaceutical companies in order to get a new drug approved for use for a given disease indication. If a cure for IBD is discovered in a laboratory where it has been developed and tested in mice, it will ultimately have to be tested in humans with IBD.

There are no wrong or right reasons for you to participate in clinical research. People participate in clinical research for a variety of reasons. Some want to have a chance to try new therapies that they normally wouldn't otherwise have access to because the therapies are not yet approved for use or because of prohibitive cost. Others want to advance research in the field so that others can benefit from the new knowledge that will be obtained from the study. Some people like the close follow-up and monitoring and quick-and-easy access to the health-care team that is typically provided as part of a clinical trial.

Questions to Ask

- What is the purpose of the study?
- Why do researchers believe the new treatment being tested may be effective?
- Has it been tested before?
- What kinds of tests and treatments are involved?
- How do the possible risks, side effects, and benefits in the study compare with my current treatment?
- What are the alternative treatments that are available to me?
- How might this trial affect my daily life?
- How long does the trial last?
- Will hospitalization be required?
- Who will pay for the treatment?
- Will I be reimbursed for other expenses, such as parking or bus fare?
- What type of long-term follow-up care is part of this study? Will I be able to receive the study medication after I have finished participating in the study?
- Will results of the trials be provided to me?
- Who will be in charge of my care?

Surgery Option

Although many patients, families, and physicians focus on medications as the primary means of treating IBD, drugs are just one aspect of the care of the patient. This care must encompass not only drug therapy, but must also address, where necessary, the nutritional and psychological aspects of the disease. In addition, surgery is a very important part of the management of IBD.

The need for surgery should not necessarily be considered a failure of the person with IBD, of their family, or of the health-care team. While recent advances in drug therapy may reduce the need for surgery in the future, surgery can provide patients in some situations with relief from symptoms that may not be possible using medications.

CHAPTER 8
Surgical Treatment of IBD

CASE STUDY Kelly

Kelly, the university student with ulcerative colitis, did very well with the drug treatment first prescribed by her specialist. She was put on prednisone and, although she did notice some swelling of her face and some weight gain, she was quite happy that her symptoms of abdominal cramps, diarrhea, urgency to move her bowels, and rectal bleeding subsided. Her prednisone dose was reduced over a period of 10 weeks and then stopped. She was placed on 5-ASA maintenance therapy to keep her well.

Although Kelly did well for 8 months, her symptoms came back with a vengeance during the following school year. Once again, she felt better with a 10-week course of prednisone, but experienced three more flares over the next 2 years, each one requiring a course of prednisone and each one improving less quickly and less completely than the flare before. The flares recurred despite Kelly being placed on the biologic drug infliximab by a gastroenterologist, and she was not able to get off prednisone without getting much worse. She continued to have very troubling side effects from the prednisone. Out of desperation, Kelly even tried a number of naturopathic remedies and probiotic treatment.

At her next appointment with her gastroenterologist, Kelly declares that she is "fed up" with her disease, with the medications, and with their side effects. She has missed several semesters of school because of her illness. She wants to get on with her life. Her gastroenterologist raises the possibility of surgery as a means of managing her disease. She knows that IBD can't be cured and wonders if surgery would be just a temporary fix. She wonders what type of surgery she would need. She also wonders if the surgery would leave her needing to have a bag to collect her stool. Will she be able to have children? She has heard that there are some newer surgical techniques that are less invasive and wonders whether she might be a candidate for one of those procedures. Her doctor was pleased to advise her on surgery options.

The Need for Surgery

Risk of Surgery

Approximately 70% to 80% of people suffering from Crohn's disease and approximately 20% to 40% of people suffering from ulcerative colitis will require surgery at some point following their diagnosis. These estimates are based on information from previous decades and do not necessarily reflect the effect of recent advances in drug therapy. There is some indication that surgical rates are coming down in coincidence with the introduction of these newer therapies. Nevertheless, there is still a substantial proportion of IBD sufferers who end up requiring surgery for their disease.

Although there are many drug therapies for treating Crohn's disease and ulcerative colitis, there are cases where this treatment does not bring symptoms under adequate control or where the side effects of the treatment are too serious or are more than the patient can tolerate. The symptoms of IBD may be so severe, come on so suddenly, or persist for so long that surgery becomes a preferred or required treatment option. There are also cases where a complication of IBD may occur that cannot be addressed adequately with drug therapy but can be resolved with surgery.

Risk and Benefit Analysis

In some of these cases, the symptoms do not improve with treatment because the disease has resulted in damage or scarring of the intestine and medications typically do not reverse most forms of damage. As a result, the IBD sufferer may never feel entirely healthy and may have significant restrictions on work and social life despite being on medication. At that point,

 Q **What does surgery involve? How long will I need to stay in the hospital?**

 A Most of the operations performed for IBD have certain features in common. First, the medical professional performing surgery will be a surgeon, usually someone other than the doctor who has been managing the other aspects of your treatment, typically a gastroenterologist (an internist with special training in treating gastrointestinal disorders). Second, most operations require one or more incisions on the abdomen in order for the surgeon to gain access to the involved areas of intestine. Third, most operations require a general anesthetic and a stay in hospital following surgery. The length of the hospital stay depends, to a large degree, on the nature of the operation, but averages somewhere between 7 to 10 days. Complications of surgery may increase the time in hospital. Finally, the time until full recovery averages 6 weeks, but this is highly dependent upon the type of operation, the patient's general health and nutritional state prior to surgery, and the patient's level of motivation.

surgery may help the person to feel healthier, with fewer restrictions on work, school, or leisure activities. Although surgery does involve some risk — both the risk that it may not be completely effective or the IBD may recur and the risk that it can result in a complication — and although surgery always involves some time away from work, school, or usual activities and always involves some degree of pain and discomfort, there comes a point where the suffering caused by the IBD is greater than these risks of surgery. Put another way, at some point, an IBD sufferer decides to accept these real and potential risks of surgery in order to have a better chance of feeling well.

Ileostomy and Colostomy

One form of surgery for IBD is an ostomy — either an ileostomy or a colostomy. "Ostomy" is the generic term for a procedure that brings an opening in the intestine out through the layers of the abdominal wall and the skin. This is sometimes referred to as a stoma.

If the last part of the small intestine (ileum) is brought out to the skin, this procedure is specifically called an ileostomy, and if the large intestine (colon) is brought out to the skin, it is called a colostomy. In both procedures, either a cut end of the intestine or a loop of intestine is brought through the skin. Where a loop is brought out, it is usually a temporary ostomy with the intention to close it or, if necessary, convert it to a permanent end ostomy. With the end ostomy, the wall of the intestine is turned out after it is brought out through the abdominal wall and its edge is sewn to the surrounding skin.

A colostomy is usually flat or flush with the surrounding skin, while an ileostomy usually sticks out half an inch to an inch above the level of the skin.

Because the stoma consists of the inner lining of the intestine, it is normally pink or red and may look painful or sore. However, the stoma has no pain-detecting nerve fibers and, as a result, is not actually painful to touch.

Because stomas do not have a valve or sphincter, there is no way to control if and when stool or gas is excreted from the stoma. As a result, a stoma requires an appliance or bag that fits over it to collect the stool and prevent soiling.

Some people delay or refuse to have surgery because they do not want to consider having an ileostomy. In some cases, this means that the person becomes sicker and sicker and more debilitated because their IBD is not adequately controlled by medications. When they finally do end up having surgery,

No Standard Procedure

There is no "standard surgery" for IBD; rather, there are a small number of operations that cover most of the situations. The exact nature of the surgery needs to be individualized in the same way that drug therapy must be individualized based on a patient's particular circumstances, the area of the GI tract affected, and the objectives of the surgery.

they may be at increased risk of complications because they have become sicker and weaker and they may have reduced immunity against infections. As a result, the healing of surgical incisions may not be as good and they are at increased risk of infections. Fortunately, for most people, the idea of having an ileostomy is worse than the reality of having an ileostomy, particularly when having the surgery that results in an ileostomy has such a significant impact on one's sense of well-being. Once the diseased bowel is removed surgically, the person typically starts to feel better, their nutritional state begins to improve, and their immunity improves.

 Q If I need surgery for IBD, does it mean that I'll need to wear a bag on my abdomen to collect my stool?

 A Surgery for IBD does not necessarily mean that you will have to wear a bag or appliance to collect stool from the stoma. In fact, most people undergoing surgery do not need to wear a bag after undergoing surgery or, if it is needed, it is most often temporary until the stoma is reversed or closed.

Crohn's vs. Colitis Procedures

Unlike medical therapy, where there is a large amount of overlap in terms of the types of medications that are effective in Crohn's disease and ulcerative colitis, the type of surgical operations that can be performed are often quite different. Distinguishing between ulcerative colitis and Crohn's disease is quite important before embarking upon most types of operation.

Surgical Procedures for Ulcerative Colitis

While the colectomy with an ileostomy was the most common operation in ulcerative colitis until the 1970s and 1980s, the ileostomy has been replaced in most cases with the pelvic pouch procedure.

Colectomy

When considering surgery, patients with ulcerative colitis have a major advantage over patients with Crohn's disease because their disease involves only the large intestine (colon): when the large intestine is surgically removed, the disease is effectively "cured."

Removing the large intestine is called a colectomy. Because the rectum is always diseased in ulcerative colitis, it has to be removed along with the rest of the large intestine; as a result, it is not possible to reattach the lower end of the small intestine to any part of the large intestine.

Ileostomy, Colostomy, Diverting Loop Ileostomy

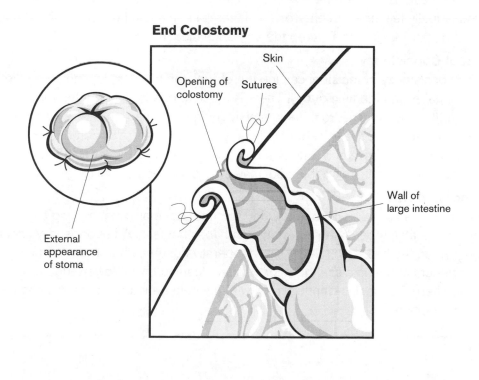

End Ileostomy

Sutures

Junction of skin and
bowel lining

Opening of
ileostomy

Wall of small
intestine

Skin

Diverting Loop Ileostomy

Opening of
ileostomy

Skin

Small intestine
(ileum)

End Colostomy

Skin

Opening of
colostomy

Sutures

Wall of
large intestine

External
appearance
of stoma

Living with a Stoma

Most people who have a stoma do very well with it and are able to adapt as necessary. There is seldom a need to change everyday activities or avoid physical activity. Competitive sports and sexual relations are possible for someone who has had the procedure performed. Immediately after surgery, the stoma may be somewhat swollen, but this will usually go down during the first 6 weeks after surgery. A stoma should almost never get in the way of leading a full and active life.

Appliances

The apparatus that attaches to the skin and that holds the bag over a stoma is known as an appliance. Several types of appliances are available, each with its own advantages and disadvantages. Patients may have to try several different appliances before finding one that works well for their build, stoma location, and lifestyle.

The assistance of an enterostomal therapy nurse (ET nurse) can be extremely valuable in avoiding frustration and in finding an appropriate appliance as quickly as possible after surgery. The ET nurse can also play an important role in the education of the IBD sufferer about the proper care and maintenance of the stoma, thereby reducing the possibility of future problems.

Self-Consciousness

People are often concerned about the appliance being obvious under clothing, but, in most instances, others will not be aware that you have a stoma unless you actually tell them. An enterostomal therapy nurse can help you with various methods or tricks to try to keep the appliance hidden.

Stool Consistency

The consistency of the stool coming out of the stoma varies depending on diet, fluid intake, and the time of day. There is a period of adaptation after surgery when the stool may go from being mainly liquid to having a thicker consistency. With an ileostomy, the stool generally gets to a consistency of porridge or toothpaste after several weeks or months, but it is almost never fully formed or solid. With a colostomy, the stool may eventually become solid.

Odor and Gas

Odor and gas are also concerns. Odor is usually not a problem as long as the appliance fits properly over the stoma and does not leak. An odor usually occurs only when the bag is emptied. This is generally done in a bathroom, and air fresheners can help mask the odor. Proper cleaning of the lower edge of the bag, where the stool is emptied from, will also help avoid odor once the bag has been emptied.

Gas may be a more difficult problem to deal with. Try to avoid air swallowing, mouth breathing, smoking, gum chewing, and drinking fizzy or carbonated drinks, which all tend to increase the amount of gas passing through the stoma into the appliance. If there is a lot of gas, it results in the bag filling up very quickly and requiring more frequent emptying.

Fluids and Electrolytes

Because patients with an ileostomy do not have a functioning colon, their ability to absorb water and electrolytes may be diminished. This is normally not a problem, but people who are chronically dehydrated may be at higher risk of certain types of kidney stones. In hot weather, when someone with an ileostomy may have increased loss of fluid and electrolytes from sweat, be sure to maintain an adequate water intake (at least 2 to 3 quarts/L per day) and to take plenty of salt with your food — or, if necessary, take salt tablets.

Intimate Relationships

Before starting sexual activity, it is important not to have a full appliance. Some people prefer to use special smaller appliances and straps or devices, which secure the appliance during sexual activity. Once again, your enterostomal therapy nurse can help you to find the right appliance for your needs. You may also find that certain activities or positions are more satisfying or more secure for you and your partner. This requires a certain amount of experimentation or trial and error.

Entering into a new sexual relationship can pose particular challenges for someone with a stoma. Although your partner may not even be aware that you have a stoma during the time that you first become acquainted, it is generally a good idea to be honest and open about the stoma before going down the path of sexual intimacy. This can be a very critical time in a relationship, usually requiring a certain degree of stability.

> **Disclosure**
>
> A stoma does not have to interfere with intimacy and sexual relations with a spouse or partner, but there is no question that it does require the understanding of the spouse or partner and often some time to adjust. You may feel "dirty" or "undesirable" on account of the stoma. Telling your partner about your concerns and fears is an important step. Your partner may also have concerns or questions that you can help answer.

The nature of the explanation that you give to your partner needs to be tailored to both of your needs, but it should usually include an indication that you had surgery for an intestinal problem and that the surgery has allowed you to recover your health to the point where you feel well enough to be sexually intimate. Your partner should also understand that, as a result of the surgery, part of your intestine has been brought out through the skin and that you have to collect the stool in a secure bag or appliance.

Before the late 1970s and early 1980s, undergoing a colectomy meant that the small intestine had to be brought through an incision in the skin as an ileostomy so that the fecal waste material would drain into an external appliance or bag. For most people with ulcerative colitis, that was the end of their problems with inflammatory bowel disease. They were able to discontinue all medications, and they felt healthy without experiencing bleeding or abdominal pain.

However, the operation left them physically changed. For many individuals, the idea of a permanent ileostomy was not easy to accept. Despite the fact that most patients adapt well to an ileostomy, it is still not what anyone would consider to be an "ideal" outcome, all other considerations aside.

Pelvic Pouch Procedure

To address the adverse personal reactions that may occur to the usual ileostomy, surgeons have developed the pelvic pouch procedure, also known as the ileal pouch-anal anastomosis (IPAA). This procedure is now offered to most patients who require a colectomy for ulcerative colitis. Elderly patients and those with damage to the anal sphincter (valve) mechanism, primarily women who have experienced damage to the sphincter during difficult or traumatic childbirth, may not be candidates for the operation. The large majority of ulcerative colitis patients who undergo the pelvic pouch procedure are pleased with the results of the operation.

In the pelvic pouch procedure, the colon and most of the rectum are removed. Then the surgeon takes the lower end of the small intestine (ileum), partially opens it up, and folds it back upon itself to fashion it into a large-capacity pouch. The pouch is then attached to the remaining very bottom part of the rectum, which is just above the anus.

In most situations, the small intestine above the pouch is brought out to the skin as a temporary ileostomy, which is reversed (closed) in a second operation 3 to 6 months later. The temporary ileostomy effectively prevents the fecal material from going through the pouch in order to allow it to heal well or, at least, to reduce the negative consequences and risk of infection if there is a problem with healing.

When a patient is very sick, poorly nourished, or on biologic medications or steroids at the time the colectomy is performed, the creation of the pouch is usually delayed until the patient is in better health, better nourished, and off steroids and biologic drugs.

High Satisfaction

The pelvic pouch procedure is offered to most patients who need surgery for ulcerative colitis. More than 90% end up being very satisfied with the result.

Gas

Although gas is not necessarily a sign of a problem with the pouch, it can be embarrassing, and the larger amounts of gas production can also cause patients to feel that they have to move their bowels more frequently than they normally would.

Pelvic (Ileal) Pouch Procedure

Panel 1

Loop ileostomy

Pelvic pouch

Remainder of rectum

The pelvic pouch procedure is usually done in two or three stages. Initially, the pouch is formed by folding the small intestine (ileum) back on itself to make a "J" shape. The bottom of the "J" is opened and sewn to the small segment of remaining rectum (detail panel). The temporary loop ileostomy is created above the pouch (panel 1), and several months later, the ileostomy is closed (panel 2), thus producing an intact digestive tract (panel 3).

Panel 2

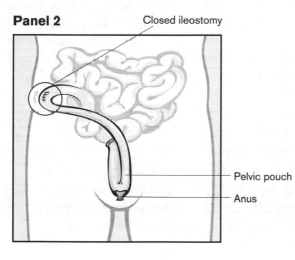

Closed ileostomy

Pelvic pouch

Anus

Detail Panel

Suturing of ileal pouch to remainder of rectum

Panel 3

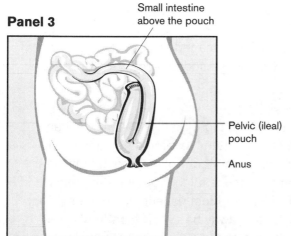

Small intestine above the pouch

Pelvic (ileal) pouch

Anus

Living with a Pelvic Pouch

Following pelvic pouch surgery and closing of the temporary ileostomy, patients usually take several weeks or months to become accustomed to the functioning of the pouch.

Bowel Movements

Patients will typically have anywhere from 4 to 12 bowel movements per day, but usually without cramps, urgency, or bleeding. The average number of bowel movements is 6 to 8 per day. The stool often has a soft or loose consistency, but may be somewhat formed in some patients. However, frequency of bowel movements can vary widely, depending on many factors, including how much fluid is being consumed and the types of food in the diet.

Stool Odor and Consistency

Many patients who have had the pelvic pouch procedure report changes in the smell of the stool and in the amount and smell of gas. The stool tends to be very irritating to the skin, and if it is not cleaned off well after a bowel motion, the skin can become red, itchy, painful, or even break down. Barrier creams containing zinc can sometimes be helpful in protecting the skin.

In some instances, the consistency of the stool and smell of the gas can be modified by adjusting the diet. Although there are certain foods that are advised against in individuals who have undergone the pelvic pouch procedure, finding foods that agree and don't agree with you is usually a matter of trial and error.

Soiling

Leakage of stool from the anus can occur following the pelvic pouch procedure. This tends to occur primarily during sleep; it is usually a minor amount leading to only some minor soiling. This can usually be managed by putting a small pad inside one's underwear or nightclothes. Regular episodes of loss of stool control during the daytime is rare.

Bowel Control

Although patients with a pelvic pouch may have more bowel movements than would be considered "normal" and the stool is often looser and perhaps even smellier than normal, the fact that they can usually control their need to move their bowels, that they no longer need medications to control their symptoms, and that they feel well offsets these inconveniences. Most patients are quite satisfied with the procedure; they are generally far and away better off than they were prior to surgery and better off than they imagine they would be with an ileostomy.

Very Loose Stools

For people with very loose or watery stools, supplementation of the diet with a source of soluble fiber, such as psyllium, may be helpful. For some individuals, antidiarrheal medications, such as loperamide (Imodium), can reduce the frequency of bowel motions enough to make them much more comfortable, particularly in social or work situations.

Complications

A number of complications of the pelvic pouch procedure can occur. Some of these are related to the operation itself — the risk of a general anesthetic, pneumonia, blood clot in the legs or lungs, and wound infection or wound opening — and go along with any type of abdominal surgery. Some of these complications are relatively minor and can be managed, but others can pose serious obstacles to patients who want to return to a normal life and good health.

Bowel Obstruction

Perhaps the most common complication is a bowel obstruction or blockage, which results in abdominal pain, nausea, vomiting, and usually a decrease in bowel motions. This can occur as soon as several days or a week following surgery and is thought to be due to adhesions (scar tissue) that form on the outside of the intestine after surgery. These adhesions can lead to kinking or twisting of the bowel, causing obstruction.

Infections

In the pelvic pouch procedure, the suturing (stitching) or stapling where the pouch is created or attached to the rectum can leak or come apart. This can lead to an abscess or serious infection in the abdominal cavity. Most pouch leaks will heal without having to operate again. However, it is important to avoid this type of complication before it occurs, because not only is it potentially serious in the short term, it also tends to lead to poorer functioning of the pouch months or years later once the leak has healed. This means that there may be more bowel motions on average, more potential leakage of stool, and possible problems with emptying the pouch.

Pouchitis

Another complication that can occur after pelvic pouch surgery is an inflammation of the inner lining of the pouch, called pouchitis. This condition occurs in approximately 10% to 15% of patients undergoing the pouch procedure, although some centers that have a large experience with the pelvic pouch procedure report higher rates of pouchitis.

Pouchitis presents with symptoms of increased stool frequency and stool looseness, abdominal cramping, loss of control of bowel motions, blood in the stool, and not feeling well.

> ### Obstruction Outcomes
>
> Bowel obstructions that occur soon after surgery usually settle down on their own after several days, but they can cause increased pain and discomfort for the patient and can lengthen the stay in hospital. If the obstruction does not settle on its own, it may require surgery to relieve it. Some individuals can also develop obstruction months or years after the pelvic pouch procedure.

> ### "Colitis" of the Pouch
>
> Acute pouchitis occurs in 10% to 15% of people undergoing the pelvic pouch procedure. In many ways, it looks and feels like ulcerative colitis of the pouch.

Treating Pouchitis

Antibiotics: Bacteria are apparently important in causing pouchitis because it almost always responds to a 7- to 14-day course of antibiotics. This is quite different from ulcerative colitis, where antibiotics are usually not effective. Ciprofloxacin (Cipro) is the antibiotic of choice for the first treatment of pouchitis, but many doctors prescribe metronidazole (Flagyl) or a combination of the two.

A small percentage of patients who recover from a first episode of pouchitis develop repeated episodes. Usually, these respond again to another course of antibiotics, but some of these patients end up having some degree of ongoing or persisting pouchitis and may require regular antibiotic treatment to keep the pouchitis under some degree of control.

Probiotics: Another approach to controlling chronic pouchitis or preventing recurrent episodes is the use of probiotics, the so-called good bacteria, such as *Lactobacillus acidophilus* and bifidobacterium, which are normally present in the human intestine. When probiotics are taken, usually in the form of a capsule or as a powder mixed with food or drink, they may have a beneficial effect on the health of the pouch by preventing recurrent episodes of pouchitis. Probiotics may also be found in some types of yogurts.

Medications: When antibiotics are not helping someone with chronic pouchitis, some of the medications that are routinely used to treat ulcerative colitis are occasionally tried. These medications are often not very helpful.

Surgery: It is rare for a patient to require surgical removal of the pelvic pouch because of chronic pouchitis and poor pouch function. In those cases, an ileostomy is usually required because there is a high chance that if a new pouch is created, similar problems will occur again.

Surgical Procedures for Crohn's Disease

Unlike ulcerative colitis, Crohn's disease can affect any part of the gastrointestinal tract and can recur in previously unaffected segments of intestine following surgical resection of a diseased area. Although there are theoretically many different types of operations that can be performed for Crohn's disease, in practice, a handful of operations account for the majority actually performed, chiefly small intestine and large intestine resections and perianal procedures.

The tendency for Crohn's disease to come back in previously unaffected segments of bowel is one of the main reasons that patients give for not wanting to undergo surgery for Crohn's disease. They worry that, after going to all of the trouble and taking on the pain and risk of surgery, they might be back at "square one" within a year or two of having undergone surgery. However, similar to the situation with ulcerative colitis, avoidance of surgery or excessive delays in going for surgery when the disease is not being adequately controlled by medications can result in progressive worsening of the patient's general status and reduced immunity. When surgery is finally carried out, this can lead to increased infections and complications and slower recovery times.

Small Intestinal Resection

The most common operation performed for Crohn's disease is a small intestinal resection. This is usually performed because an area of small intestine is affected by Crohn's disease, and this has led to scarring and narrowing of the intestinal opening through which food passes. This produces symptoms of pain, bloating, nausea, and vomiting after meals and can even lead to bowel obstruction. Small intestinal resections may also be required when a fistula or an abscess has arisen from an affected segment of intestine or when symptoms of active inflammation in the small intestine (abdominal cramping, diarrhea, weight loss) do not respond to drug therapies.

Ileocecal Resection

When the large intestine has no obvious Crohn's disease, only the very first part of the colon, called the cecum, is resected. This is called an ileocecal resection: the last part of the ileum and the first part of the colon are taken out together as a single piece of intestine.

> **Recurrence**
>
> Whereas removal of the large intestine in ulcerative colitis leads to a "cure" with no chance of ulcerative colitis recurring in the small intestine or other parts of the gastrointestinal tract, Crohn's disease can recur in previously unaffected segments of intestine following surgical resection of a diseased area. This may lead to the need for multiple operations and removal of additional intestinal segments at each operation.

Q   What is short bowel syndrome?

A   The surgical approach to Crohn's disease may require several different procedures and several repetitions of the same procedure. Ultimately, this can result in the removal of so much intestine that it leaves patients unable to keep themselves nourished and to maintain fluid and electrolyte balance through the intake of food and liquids. This condition, called short bowel syndrome, is a serious consequence of Crohn's disease surgery and can lead to the need for long-term or permanent intravenous feeding at home (home total parenteral nutrition, or HTPN).

To avoid this, there is a tendency, where it is safe, to delay surgery for Crohn's disease, and when surgery is needed, the surgeon will usually try to resect only the minimum amount of bowel necessary to deal with the immediate problem.

Extent of Resection

Although any part of the small intestine can be affected with Crohn's disease, the most common section is the last part of the small intestine (terminal ileum) just before the small intestine joins the large intestine. Because the diseased bowel and associated narrowing usually extends right up to the junction between the small and large intestine (ileocecal valve), it is technically impossible for the surgeon to remove just the small intestine, making it necessary to remove the ileocecal valve and an adjacent portion of the large intestine. The amount of large intestine resected is determined by whether or not it, too, is affected.

Ileocolic Resection

If part of the large intestine is affected by Crohn's disease — most commonly on the right side in an area involving the cecum and part of the ascending colon — then it is often resected along with the terminal ileum. This operation is called an ileocolic resection.

Small Intestinal Resection

When there is a normal segment of small intestine between the lowermost extent of the affected small intestine and the ileocecal valve, it is technically possible to remove only the affected segment of small intestine and not remove any of the large intestine. This is called a small intestinal resection.

Anastomosis

In all of these operations, the removal of a segment of intestine leaves two unattached, or open, ends of small intestine or one open end of small intestine and one of large intestine. These ends are sewn or stapled together to reestablish the continuous flow of intestinal contents all the way through the gastrointestinal tract.

However, in some situations, the surgeon may decide to create a temporary stoma above the surgical hookup site (anastomosis) in order to divert the intestinal contents away from the anastomosis so that it has the best chance of healing fully. This is usually done when there has been an abscess or uncontrolled infection in the area of the anastomosis prior to surgery and the risk of poor healing is higher. In most cases, the stoma is closed during another surgical procedure several months later.

Strictureplasty

Patients who have had multiple previous intestinal resections or who have multiple segments of affected small intestine are at risk of developing short bowel syndrome if they have more of their bowel removed surgically. A strictureplasty is a method of avoiding removal of additional segments of intestine. There are a number of methods of performing strictureplasty, but they all involve opening up the affected and narrowed segment of the

Strictureplasty

Narrowed section

Incision

The narrow segment of the intestine has an incision made along its length and is then sewn across to widen the opening.

Sewn together

Seton

Fistula tract (outside opening)   Seton   Anus

Abscess Drainage

Skin   Internal opening to abscess   Perianal abscess drainage intestine and creating a larger internal passageway for food to pass through without causing symptoms of obstruction.

Strictureplasty is not always done whenever there is a narrowed segment of small intestine, for several reasons. The affected segment is often too long — multiple short segments of narrowing are ideal for strictureplasty. The segment is sometimes too diseased and thickened, making it difficult to work with surgically. There may be only a single short segment of narrowing, and the risk of the strictureplasty procedure (leak, infection, recurrent obstruction) is not worth the potential benefit of avoiding a resection, which is generally much easier to perform. In the situation where the affected segment is very short, then resection of that segment carries very little risk of complication or of future development of short bowel syndrome.

Large Intestinal Resection (Colectomy)

Removal of all or part of the large intestine is less commonly done in Crohn's disease than is a small intestinal resection. It is typically performed when all or part of the colon is affected with Crohn's disease and the symptoms cannot be controlled with medication. Occasionally, the operation is performed because of one or more strictures in the colon or because of a fistula or abscess arising out of the colon.

There are a few common segments of colon that may be removed, and each of these operations has its own name describing the part of the colon that has been removed: the right half of the colon in a right hemicolectomy, the left half of the colon in a left hemicolectomy, and the sigmoid colon in a sigmoid resection.

Partial Colectomy

When a colectomy is performed, it may be partial or complete. In a partial colectomy, only a portion of the large intestine is removed and usually the two cut ends of the intestine are sewn together.

Subtotal Colectomy

A subtotal colectomy involves removal of all of the large intestine, with the exception of the rectum and perhaps the lower end of the sigmoid colon. In this operation, the last part of the small intestine (ileum) is connected to the rectum to form an ileorectal anastomosis or to the sigmoid colon to form an ileosigmoid anastomosis.

Pelvic Pouch Option

Most surgeons who perform the pelvic pouch procedure will offer the operation to a patient who appears to have ulcerative colitis, but in whom Crohn's disease cannot be absolutely ruled out, as long as there are no abscesses, fistulas, or ulcers in or around the anus, there is no evidence of a problem with function of the anal sphincter, and the patient understands that there is a higher risk of pouch failure.

Total Proctocolectomy

If the entire colon and rectum are removed, the operation is called a total proctocolectomy. The end of the small intestine is usually brought out to the skin as an ileostomy. Patients with known Crohn's disease are usually not candidates for pelvic pouch reconstruction surgery, except in special circumstances.

Pelvic Pouch Surgery

Ulcerative colitis does not recur once the rectum and colon have been removed, but Crohn's disease can come back in the pouch and in the small intestine above the pouch if the patient has undergone the pelvic pouch surgery. This frequently leads to poor pouch function, medical complications, and a very unhappy patient who has gone through several operations with the expectation of being "cured."

> **Only in Select Circumstances**
>
> If someone has Crohn's disease involving the rectum and colon, the pelvic pouch procedure is usually not offered as an option, except in very select circumstances.

Mistaken Ulcerative Colitis

Although pelvic pouch procedures are, in most circumstances, not offered to patients with known Crohn's disease, there are some patients who, despite extensive examination and investigation prior to surgery, are thought to have ulcerative colitis but subsequently are discovered to have Crohn's disease. This can occur once the entire colon has been removed and examined under a microscope by a pathologist or after being followed for many years after surgery and found ultimately to develop features of Crohn's disease, such as ulcers in the small intestine above the pouch.

In these cases, the patient with Crohn's disease is left with a pelvic pouch. Antibiotics, steroids, and immunosuppressants may be tried in this situation, but most gastroenterologists will opt for a TNF-alpha blocker biologic therapy, such as infliximab or adalimumab, as the best option to try to salvage the pouch and avoid the need for further surgery and removal of the pouch. Nevertheless, a significant proportion of patients

Small and Large Intestine Resection

Small intestine resection

Resection margins

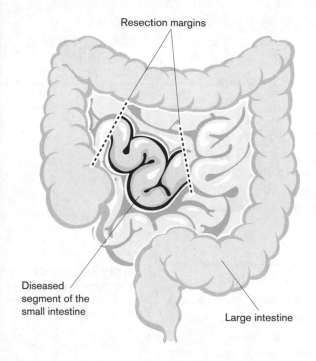

Diseased
segment of the
small intestine

Large intestine

Margins sewn together

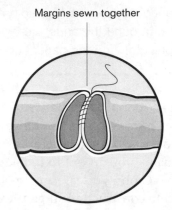

When a resection is performed,
the diseased segment of intestine
is cut out and the remaining
margins are sewn together.

Large intestine resection

Resection margins

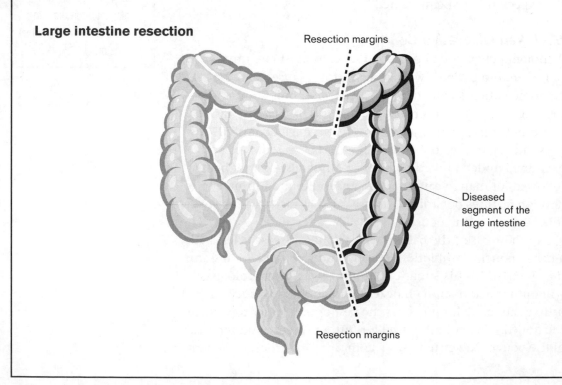

Diseased
segment of the
large intestine

Resection margins

Mapping Fistulas and Abscesses

Many operations for perianal Crohn's disease are preceded by investigations to help map out where the fistulas, if present, communicate with the rectum or with each other and to look for any abscesses that may be present but not suspected by the usual examination that can be performed in the clinic.

Physical Examinations and Tests

The usual examination involves visually inspecting the area around the anus, feeling the area around the anus, and using a finger to feel inside the anus and rectum. Other investigations include CT scan, MRI, and endoanal ultrasound. Endoanal ultrasound involves putting an ultrasound probe into the anus and rectum. The probe emits a high-frequency sound wave that bounces off the tissues and back to the probe. These sound waves are detected by the probe and converted into images on a screen. Which investigation is performed really depends on what is available at a given center and the expertise of the doctors performing the tests.

Surgical Examination

The surgery for perianal disease almost always involves an examination by the surgeon once the patient has been put under a general anesthetic (examination under anesthesia). The muscles in the area are all relaxed once the patient has received a general anesthetic, and this allows a better examination with probing of the fistula openings. The examination under anesthesia may actually help map out the disease as well as, or in some cases better than, the tests discussed above.

with Crohn's disease and a pelvic pouch — somewhere around 1 in 4 — will end up requiring further surgery and very possibly surgical removal of the pouch, with the creation of a permanent ileostomy.

Indeterminate Colitis

In some cases when IBD involves only the colon, Crohn's disease cannot be differentiated from ulcerative colitis, even when the entire colon has been removed and examined by a pathologist. In that situation, called indeterminate colitis, the pelvic pouch procedure may be offered to patients with the understanding that some will ultimately turn out to have Crohn's disease, with a higher chance of failure of the pouch procedure. However, when all patients with indeterminate colitis undergoing the pelvic pouch procedure are compared to patients with ulcerative colitis, patients with indeterminate colitis have only a slightly higher risk of pouch failure.

Perianal Surgeries

Unlike the surgery for treatment of Crohn's disease involving the intestine, surgery for the complications of Crohn's disease in the area of the anus (perianal disease) does not usually involve removing any segments of bowel.

Most operations are performed to reduce the symptoms of the perianal disease — most often pain and drainage of pus or stool — when the symptoms have not responded to other measures, such as sitz baths, antibiotics, immunosuppressants, and infliximab or adalimumab, or when an acute problem, such as an abscess, has occurred.

Incision and Drainage

Once the surgeon has adequately mapped out the extent of abscesses or fistulas, a procedure is chosen to reduce or eliminate the patient's symptoms. In some cases, this may involve cutting open the skin near the anus in order to allow an abscess to drain (incision and drainage).

Fistulotomy

In other cases, where there is a single fistula that does not cut across the anal sphincter, the surgeon may open up the fistula with an incision along its length (fistulotomy). This, in turn, allows the fistula to heal from the inside out, thereby eliminating the fistula tract.

Seton

Where there are multiple fistulas or when the fistula crosses the anal sphincter, a fistulotomy is not possible because of the likelihood of causing damage to the sphincter, which would result in problems with loss of control of the bowels (incontinence).

Instead, the surgeon may pass a string, thread, or thin plastic band through the outside opening of the fistula on the skin around the anus, along the fistula tract as it passes under the skin and toward the anus or rectum, through the internal opening of the fistula inside the anus or rectum, and back out through the anal canal. The two ends of the string are tied together, effectively creating a loop through the fistula and the anus. This string or tube, also known as a seton, keeps the fistula open and allows it to drain in a controlled way.

This result would seem to be the opposite of one of the objectives of treating perianal disease — that is, reducing drainage from the fistula. However, in many patients with fistulas, the openings of the fistulas periodically close up, thereby causing the pus that normally drains out to collect

---

Seton Option

For a person who keeps developing recurrent abscesses, a seton is a preferable option. Although it may be associated with some local irritation and drainage, it is usually minor compared to the pain that can occur when an abscess forms.

inside. This, in turn, causes more inflammation in the tissues around the fistula and the anus, and an abscess can form. Anyone who has ever had a perianal abscess knows that it is exquisitely painful and can interfere with simple activities, such as sitting, walking, and sleeping. It can also become acutely painful during a bowel motion.

The abscess must then be drained by a surgeon or, in many instances, will go away once the fistula tract has opened again on its own. Recurrent inflammation in the perianal area can lead to scarring and damage, thus making it more difficult for the area to eventually heal.

Surgical Flap

Occasionally, surgeons may attempt to repair or close off the internal opening of a fistula where it comes through inside the anus or rectum. This is most often tried when the fistula connects the rectum and the vagina. The surgical procedure involves taking a flap of tissue that is partially cut out of the inner lining of the rectum and pulling it down and over the opening of the fistula that exists inside the rectum. The flap is sewn over the opening in an attempt to keep it in place. Other methods of closing fistulas have been tried. One of these involves injecting a substance that forms a gel-like plug into the outside opening of the fistula. There have been some reports of

---

Failure Rate

Surgical flap operations, which, under the best of circumstances, have a fairly high failure rate of approximately 40% to 50%, should be attempted only if the rectum is free of active Crohn's disease and should be performed only by a surgeon experienced in the management of Crohn's disease fistulas.

Combined Approach

An approach that is often used to manage perianal Crohn's disease is a combined surgical and medical approach, whereby the surgeon drains any abscesses and puts in setons as necessary and the gastroenterologist treats the Crohn's disease with medication, most often infliximab or adalimumab. Although there haven't been large trials to study this combined approach, it appears that it may provide long-term healing and symptom control better than what can be provided by either surgery or drug therapy alone.

In addition, if a patient has active intestinal disease with resulting diarrhea, this will tend to aggravate the symptoms of the perianal disease. If drug treatment is effective in healing the intestinal lining and reducing diarrhea, this alone will have a noticeable and beneficial effect on the perianal disease.

Unfortunately, this type of combined approach is not readily available everywhere because in some areas the surgeons and gastroenterologists may not work closely together or they may not have the necessary expertise and experience in dealing with this complicated form of Crohn's disease.

good results with this technique, but it cannot be considered a standard practice until more experience has accumulated and better results have been demonstrated.

Stem Cell Therapy

A new approach to the treatment of perianal fistulas is the use of stem cells. Many people know of stem cell therapy's use in treating different types of cancers. In the case of Crohn's disease fistulas, the stem cells are used because of their potential to develop into cells that can produce factors that lead to tissue healing and closure of fistula tracts.

The stem cells are injected into the inside and outside openings of the fistulas by a surgeon during an examination under anesthesia. This therapy has been approved for use in the European Union, but continues to undergo clinical testing to determine if it really is effective and safe.

Diverting Loop (Temporary) Ileostomy

For patients with severe perianal fistulas who do not respond to these measures or who have had damage to the anal sphincter, a diverting loop (temporary) ileostomy may be the operation that provides them with the best outcome.

By preventing stool from passing through the anus and the area of the fistulas and abscesses, this particular operation may result in a reduction in drainage from the fistulas, reduced abscess formation, and, in some cases, healing of the fistulas or surgical wounds left behind after drainage of an abscess. In those instances, the ileostomy may be reversed, or closed, and the fistulas will sometimes, but not always, remain healed.

End Ileostomy

For the patients with anal sphincter damage, closure of the ileostomy may not be feasible because incontinence will occur or the fistulas and abscesses may recur. In these cases, the loop ileostomy may be converted to a more permanent end ileostomy once the affected individual becomes accustomed to having a stoma. This type of ileostomy usually functions somewhat better than the temporary type and is easier for the individual to care for.

Removal of Rectum

When the rectum is left behind and not used for many years, there appears to be risk of cancer of the rectum. This can be difficult or impossible to screen for, and diagnosis usually occurs late and after the chance for cure has passed. As a result, most surgeons and gastroenterologists recommend that the

Reducing Cancer Risk

If patients have had an end ileostomy for the treatment of rectal and perianal disease, it is usually recommended that they eventually have the rectum and anus removed surgically and the area closed up to reduce the risk of cancer of the rectum.

Laparoscopic Surgery

rectum be removed electively before cancer has had a chance to develop. This is best done once the patient's nutritional state has improved and stabilized and once the patient is off medications, such as prednisone.

Laparoscopic Surgery

Since approximately 1990, laparoscopic surgery has been used for many different types of gastrointestinal disorders, such as gallbladder disease and appendicitis. This type of surgery, sometimes referred to as minimal access surgery or keyhole surgery, involves using instruments that are passed through several (usually three or four) small incisions on the abdomen. One of the instruments is a camera that allows the surgeon to see inside the abdomen without opening it up with a large incision. The other instruments act as the "hands" of the surgeon, used for cutting, suturing, stapling, and all of the other things that a surgeon would normally do during a standard open-approach operation.

When a piece of an organ, such as the intestine, is removed, the incision at the belly button is usually extended a few centimeters to allow the intestine to be brought out. The advantage of the laparoscopic approach is that it leaves very small scars on the abdomen. These are often not noticeable unless one closely examines the area. In addition, it appears to reduce, to some extent, but does not eliminate the pain after surgery and allows faster discharge from hospital. For some operations, such as gallbladder, it allows quicker recovery and return to work or school.

Limitations

Even when a laparoscopic approach is planned when an operation is started, it is not always possible to complete the entire operation this way because there may be many adhesions (scars) within the abdomen from previous surgery that make it impossible to see well enough using the laparoscopic camera. In other cases, the Crohn's disease is too complex, with many internal fistulas from one segment of intestine to another or an abscess associated with an inflamed segment of intestine. Using a laparoscopic approach in this case would be unsafe. When surgeons encounter these limitations and complications, they will convert to an open approach.

Although laparoscopic surgery can result in major reductions in pain, hospital stay, and recovery time, these benefits over the open approach in the average case of IBD are not as obvious. There is still postoperative pain requiring medication, a hospital stay that averages about 5 days if no complications occur, and 3 to 6 weeks before someone is ready to return to work, school, and other daily activities.

Preventing Recurrence

Surgery can be a very effective way of managing your Crohn's disease. However, Crohn's disease can come back in parts of the intestine that were previously not affected. As a result, it is not unheard of for people with Crohn's disease to require two, three, four, or even more operations.

If you have had multiple operations and if a large part of your intestine has been taken out, you may ultimately not be able to adequately absorb nutrients, water, minerals, and electrolytes from your diet. This can be a very serious problem — more serious than the Crohn's disease itself. At the end of the day, the real challenge in the field of surgery for Crohn's disease is not so much how to perform an operation, but how to prevent the disease from coming back after the diseased bowel has been removed.

However, it appears that some individuals are at lower risk of recurrent Crohn's disease and may not need treatment after surgery. Unfortunately, there is no good way to predict who is at high risk and who is at relatively low risk.

Stop Smoking

Perhaps the best way to reduce the risk of recurrence of Crohn's disease after surgery is not to smoke cigarettes. Although it has not been proven that for smokers who quit after surgery the risk of recurrent disease is lower, it has been shown that smokers tend to have earlier and more severe recurrences after surgery. So, if you don't already smoke, don't start after surgery, and if you do smoke, consider attempting to quit. Not only will this benefit your Crohn's disease, but it will have other health benefits (reduced heart disease, lower cancer risk, less lung disease).

Medications

Some patients, particularly those who have had a very short segment of intestine removed or who had disease for many years before coming to surgery, may choose not to take medication following surgery. For some patients, one goal in undergoing surgery is to stop medication, and this needs to be considered when discussing the management of Crohn's disease after surgery.

Although the 5-ASA medications are probably the safest and best tolerated, they have a very modest effect on the risk of recurrence, reducing the risk of recurrence by about 10% to 12%. Metronidazole and other related antibiotics also appear to reduce recurrence, but not all patients are able to tolerate the medications because of a metallic taste in the mouth and gastrointestinal upset. It is not clear whether the beneficial effect of antibiotics extends past 1 year after surgery.

The immunosuppressants azathioprine and 6-mercaptopurine are being used more often for prevention of recurrence after surgery for Crohn's disease, despite the fact that the evidence supporting their use is not entirely clear. Nevertheless, there is a sense among expert IBD physicians that these drugs are among the best maintenance treatments available and, if monitored properly, have good safety records. These drugs are used particularly when a person has had very severe or complicated disease prior to surgery, if a relatively long length of intestine has been surgically removed, or if it is not the first operation for Crohn's disease.

Infliximab has been shown to be effective for the treatment of acute flares of Crohn's disease as well as maintenance therapy. Because of its effectiveness in those situations, there has also been interest in using infliximab after surgery. There is some evidence that it is an effective preventive treatment after surgery, but it still remains to be determined which patients would benefit most from its use.

> ### Drug Effectiveness
>
> A number of different medications have been tried as a way to reduce the risk of recurrent Crohn's disease after surgery. None of the currently available drugs is 100% effective. The ones most commonly used are 5-aminosalicylic acid (5-ASA) containing preparations, antibiotics, and azathioprine or 6-mercaptopurine (6-MP). These are all discussed in more detail in the chapter on drug therapy.

Follow-Up Colonoscopy and Medications

In an effort to determine which patients to recommend for preventive treatment after surgery, particularly for treatment with an immunosuppressant drug, such as azathioprine or 6-mercaptopurine, or an antitumor necrosis factor drug, such as infliximab or adalimumab, many gastroenterologists are conducting a colonoscopy at some point in the first 12 months after surgery. It is well known that early signs seen by colonoscopy can occur well before symptoms of Crohn's disease recur, and this provides an opportunity to treat the Crohn's disease before the lesions progress to more severe types of lesions, which can then frequently result in symptoms and complications. Patients who develop these lesions within the first year after surgery are at higher risk for having more progressive or aggressive disease recurrence, and they are then offered the opportunity to go on drug therapy or, if they are already on drug therapy, to adjust or change their therapy to get better control of the disease.

Children with IBD

These concerns about surgery, drug therapy, and recurrence of IBD are especially important when treating children with Crohn's disease and ulcerative colitis. Parents play a vital role in translating this complex information to their children, while helping them to make the "right" decision for treatment.

CASE STUDY Lauren

Lauren is a 26-year-old woman who works for an advertising agency. She has had Crohn's disease for 7 years. She first visited her doctor with symptoms of abdominal pain and diarrhea, but had no fatigue, loss of appetite, or weight loss. She had several painful reddish-purple lumps on her shins, which her gastroenterologist told her were a feature of Crohn's disease called erythema nodosum.

Lauren was treated with budesonide and methotrexate, and while she improved, she wasn't able to stop taking budesonide without her symptoms coming back. Eventually, she started taking a TNF-alpha blocker and did very well; she was then able to stop the budesonide and remained well.

When she graduated from university, however, she was no longer covered under her mother's drug insurance plan, and she missed about 9 months of TNF-alpha blocker therapy while coverage under the public drug insurance plan was being arranged. Toward the end of that time, her symptoms started to come back even though she was still taking methotrexate.

Although she resumed taking the TNF-alpha blocker once her coverage resumed, her symptoms did not improve and she was actually experiencing even worse pain that seemed to come on after every meal and would last for several hours. This was associated with nausea and a feeling of being bloated, and she occasionally vomited.

Her gastroenterologist increased the dose of her TNF-alpha blocker, with no apparent results. He suggested further testing, since Lauren was obviously not doing well. A colonoscopy showed no signs of Crohn's disease in the colon, but an MRI scan of the small intestine (MR enterography) showed a 4-inch (10 cm) segment of thickening in the last part of the small intestine (the terminal ileum). The internal channel of the intestine in that thickened segment was quite narrow, but it looked like most of the thickening and narrowing was due to fibrosis (scar tissue). There appeared to be very little swelling that was caused by inflammation.

Lauren is now back at her gastroenterologist's clinic to review the test results and plan further management of her disease. She has recently gotten engaged, and the wedding is in 8 months. She and her fiancé plan to start a family within a couple of years. Lauren brings up all of these considerations in her discussions with her doctor.

Her gastroenterologist tells her there are other biologic drugs she could try, but he is not highly confident that they will have a major impact on her symptoms at this point, since most of what she is experiencing is due to scarring. Since the Crohn's disease is limited to a relatively short segment of small intestine, he tells Lauren that she will likely have a very good outcome from surgery. Although there is always a chance that Crohn's disease can come back after surgery, the surgery will likely get her several years of good health, during which she can get married and have children, possibly without even being on medication.

Lauren is quite interested in the surgical option and asks for a referral to a colorectal surgeon.

CHAPTER 9
Treating Children with IBD

CASE STUDY Michael

Michael is a 14-year-old boy who has always been a good student. He has been popular and active in sports, especially hockey. Over the past year or so, he has experienced occasional episodes of abdominal pain and diarrhea. These have usually lasted only a few days, going away on their own. Although Michael missed a day or two of school and sports activities during these episodes, they did not occur often and his parents did not think much about them.

However, Michael noticed that most of the boys on his hockey team were getting much bigger and were going through puberty, whereas he had not experienced the growth spurt, deepening of the voice, and body hair growth that his friends had experienced. The size difference made it more difficult to compete in hockey. He was also feeling more tired than usual.

When he paid his annual visit to his pediatrician, Michael was routinely weighed and measured. His doctor pointed out that his rate of linear growth (height) had fallen off over the last 2 years. Previously, he was at the 50th percentile for his age — in other words, he had been just about average — but now he was at the 10th percentile, meaning that approximately 90% of boys his age are taller than him. The pediatrician was concerned with this growth delay, as well as Michael's fatigue and abdominal symptoms.

She decided to order some blood tests and an ultrasound scan of the abdomen. The blood tests showed anemia and iron deficiency, and the ultrasound showed an 8-inch (20 cm) segment of small intestine that appeared thickened and inflamed, possibly due to Crohn's disease. She referred Michael to a pediatric gastroenterologist, who carried out a colonoscopy and then discussed the treatment options with Michael and his parents.

Available treatments included both drug treatment (steroids, immunosuppressives, biologic drugs), nutritional therapy, and surgery. After much discussion of the pros and cons, Michael and his parents elected to try nutritional therapy with feeding of a liquid nutritional supplement through a nasogastric tube and iron supplementation. Michael was taught to place the tube himself through his nose and into his stomach each evening and remove it each morning. During the daytime, he primarily took a fluid diet, but occasionally had some favorite food — french fries, potato chips, or other snack foods — when he was with his friends. After several months of therapy, Michael's energy level improved and he was not experiencing any more episodes of abdominal pain and diarrhea. His checkup at 3 months indicated that he had grown an inch (2.5 cm) and was showing some signs of entering puberty.

Family Challenges

Crohn's disease and ulcerative colitis are two chronic disorders that commonly affect children. If you are the parent of a child with IBD, you will know that the management of the disease in your child presents special challenges. The disease can cause great strain within the family unit, and even the strongest families may find it difficult to cope with the stress of having a child with a chronic illness for which there is no cure. This can be particularly difficult when children are very young and do not know what is happening to them. Trying to explain to children why they are not feeling well is never easy.

Parents may find it more difficult to cope with the symptoms, medications, hospitalizations, and prospect of possible surgery associated with their child's disease than the child does. For the most part, children tend to be very resilient and adapt well to new situations and new challenges, especially when given appropriate support. The support of parents, other family members, and the health-care team can help the child meet the challenges ahead. The support of friends and teachers is also important.

> **Childhood Risk**
>
> Approximately 20% of individuals with IBD develop the disease when they are children or adolescents. IBD is very uncommon in infants and toddlers, but the incidence gradually increases during childhood and adolescence.

Special Management

Although Crohn's disease and ulcerative colitis in children are similar in many ways to IBD in adults, the way the disease presents and the way it is managed require special consideration.

Disease Type

When inflammatory bowel disease is recognized in very young children, under 5 years of age, the inflammation is usually in the colon. This colitis could be either chronic ulcerative colitis or Crohn's colitis. In very young children, the appearance of the disease in the colon is not as well defined as in teenagers and adults, making it harder to distinguish the type of colitis.

Outside of the preschool age group, the percentage of children and teenagers with Crohn's disease or ulcerative colitis is similar to the percentage observed among adults in the same geographic region. In North America, for example, Crohn's disease occurs more commonly than ulcerative colitis in adults and in older children and teenagers.

Intestinal Location

The locations of the disease in the intestinal tract are somewhat different in children than in adults, although there is a large degree of overlap. In children with ulcerative colitis, the disease most commonly involves the entire colon (pancolitis or extensive colitis), whereas, in adults, up to 50% of ulcerative colitis sufferers will have inflammation limited to the last part of the colon and rectum.

In children with Crohn's disease, just as in adults, different parts of the intestinal tract can be inflamed. Apart from the very youngest children, the percentage of children and adolescents with small intestine, large intestine, and combined small and large intestine involvement with Crohn's disease seem to be similar to that of adults. Involvement of the upper part of the small intestine (jejunum) is not common in children (occurs in less than 10%), but it may be more common in children than in adults.

Growth and Development

Chronic diseases in children may affect growth and development. Not only the disease itself but also the treatments can pose problems.

Disease Effects

Inflammatory bowel disease itself can have a very important negative effect on growth, even before the disease is diagnosed.

Catch Up

Although the inflammation associated with IBD can result in a reduced rate of growth, adequate treatment of the IBD, whether through the appropriate use of medications, nutritional supplements, or surgical treatment, can allow a child to have some degree of "catch-up" growth. The rate of growth increases to a rate above normal so that the child, in effect, catches up to a height close to what it was destined to be before IBD developed. The target height, of course, is generally reflected by the parents' heights.

However, there is only limited opportunity for catch-up growth. Once the child reaches a certain age — which varies from child to child — further catch-up growth is no longer possible and the child may not attain the maximum possible height. For example, girls usually finish growing in height within 2 years of their first menstrual period. Boys generally enter puberty and finish growing on average 2 years later than girls.

A child can experience poor growth for several years before Crohn's disease is recognized and treated.

A falloff in growth rate that occurs before a child develops symptoms, such as abdominal pain or diarrhea, may be very puzzling for the pediatrician and parent. The reason may become apparent only once other symptoms develop and a diagnosis of IBD is made. This effect on growth is much more commonly seen in Crohn's disease than in ulcerative colitis. The reasons for the difference are not well understood.

Drug Side Effects

Historically, many of the treatments used in adults have also been used in children, sometimes without solid proof that these treatments are as effective in children as they are in adults. Not all drugs commonly used in adults are necessarily desirable to use in children because of their potential for side effects and the concerns about long-term safety or delayed effects that may be observed many years after the drug is taken.

Steroids

Steroid medications, such as prednisone, are very effective at reducing the intestinal inflammation in both Crohn's disease and ulcerative colitis, and, as a result, they can improve symptoms, such as abdominal pain, diarrhea, and rectal bleeding. However, in children, they also have the potential to reduce growth noticeably, if they are used for extended periods.

Immunosuppressants

In Crohn's disease, there has been a tendency to use immunosuppressive medications, such as azathioprine, 6-mercaptopurine, or methotrexate, whenever a child requires steroids to bring their disease symptoms under control. When effective, these drugs will allow the child to taper off the steroid without relapsing and will reduce the need for further courses of steroids over a period of several years. This avoidance of steroids may be very important in allowing the child to grow normally and reach full height potential.

Biologic Drugs

The newer targeted, or "designer," biologic drugs have been increasingly used to treat children with IBD, particularly those who have more severe disease and those who are not able to avoid the use of steroid medications. The TNF-alpha blockers are the most commonly used biologic drugs in children, and they have been found to be highly effective and as safe as or safer than steroids or immunosuppressants such as

> **Steroid Care**
>
> Doctors who treat children with Crohn's disease and ulcerative colitis will prescribe steroid medications for a significant flare-up of IBD, but they are careful to avoid long-term use of steroids, recognizing that this would have negative effects on growth.

azathioprine or 6-mercaptopurine. The TNF-alpha blockers do not interfere with growth; in fact, when they effectively control inflammation, they can result in increased growth.

So far, after 20 or more years of use, the long-term safety of these drugs appears to be good. There is not nearly as much experience with the use in children of the more recently introduced biologic drugs vedolizumab and ustekinumab, but so far there have been no major surprises with respect to differences between how children and adults react to these drugs. However, much more work needs to be done to adequately assure both the effectiveness and the safety of the newer biologic drugs in children.

Delayed Puberty

A slowing of growth in height is usually associated with a delay in pubertal development as well. Keeping pace with the growth and development of one's friends can be very important to the self-esteem of a child with IBD. When a child's friends are growing rapidly and developing the physical characteristics of a mature woman or man, the child with IBD may still have the stature and appearance of a younger child. This can make it very difficult for the children to fit in with their peers and, unfortunately, can make it more likely that they will become the target of teasing or even bullying. Physical-appearance problems may be compounded by the effect of a medication, such as prednisone, which can cause delayed growth, weight gain, and rounding of the face.

Inflammatory Proteins

Growth delay and the associated delay in pubertal development result from a number of different but interrelated factors. The most important factors seem to be inflammatory proteins produced by the diseased bowel. These proteins can have many effects, including reduction of appetite and thus food intake, and interference with growth-hormone pathways. Controlling the activity of the disease through the appropriate use of medications or surgery, avoiding certain medications, such as steroids, and maintaining good nutrition can help to optimize a child's growth.

Irregular Periods

Once a girl has reached puberty and menstrual cycles have started, it is not uncommon for her to experience irregular periods or even to have her period stop, particularly when she is experiencing a disease flare. Encourage your daughter to bring this issue to the attention of her doctor, because irregular or

---

Treatment Goal

Facilitating normal growth and pubertal development is a major treatment goal. Parents should be encouraged to advocate for treatments that will enhance growth rather than further inhibiting it. If your child's self-esteem is affected by delayed growth and pubertal development, you should bring this to the attention of the health-care team.

---

absent menstrual periods may interfere with her developing strong bones. This, in turn, may lead to an increased risk of osteoporosis later in life.

Long-Term Treatment

Both Crohn's disease and ulcerative colitis are chronic disorders that cannot be cured by medical or nutritional therapy. Although surgery can be "curative" for ulcerative colitis, it is not a perfect solution because of early and late complications.

For every drug developed for the treatment of IBD, there are concerns about the delayed or long-term consequences of being on the medication, particularly if it is used continuously and if it is used from an early age. These effects cannot always be predicted based on our knowledge of how the drug works, and they may not be apparent for many years after the drug is available for general use. As a result, the use of any new medication for the treatment of IBD is likely to involve a certain amount of risk-taking, particularly when used in children.

An area of specific concern in children is the use of immunosuppressive medications. Although this class of medications has a very good safety record, they do, as their name suggests, suppress the body's immune system to a certain extent and, as a result, can lead to a slightly increased risk of infections. In addition, there is some evidence to suggest that azathioprine and 6-mercaptopurine (6-MP) result in a slightly increased risk of lymphoma (cancer of the lymph glands).

This cancer is quite uncommon. Even for individuals taking azathioprine or 6-MP, the risk is still very small — probably somewhere in the range of 1 in 5,000 to 1 in 10,000. The risk does appear to be somewhat higher in young males, and there is one particularly aggressive form of lymphoma, hepatosplenic T-cell lymphoma, that seems to occur almost exclusively in young males treated with azathioprine or 6-MP. Many IBD patients and their families are willing to accept these small potential risks, particularly if there is immediate benefit to be had by being on the medications.

Psychological Issues

For parents, it's tough enough raising a child without having to deal with a chronic illness such as IBD. The addition of IBD to the mix creates some special psychological challenges to the parent–child relationship.

Parenting Styles

Different parents have different ways of reacting to illness in a child. There is no absolute wrong or right way of interacting

> ### Important Considerations
>
> Although the long-term effects of treatments for the disease, especially drug treatments, are important considerations in adults with IBD, they are even more important in children.

> ### Positive Parenting Attitudes
>
> - Your child may have inflammatory bowel disease, but this does not mean that you love or value your child any less.
> - Your child is not at fault for having developed IBD.
> - You are not at fault for your child having developed IBD.
> - Your child has not disappointed you.

with a child with a chronic disease as long as a supportive and caring environment is maintained. IBD is a challenge that should be approached together as a family.

Growing Independence

Working with a child with IBD depends on the age of the child. In younger children, parents have to take a very active role in the monitoring and management of the disease. However, this should be done in a supportive way so as not to be intrusive or smothering. Children should have enough "room" to become independent over time, eventually taking an active role in managing their disease.

Team Approach

Taking a "team" approach with children, whereby they are given a certain degree of defined responsibility for monitoring and managing their disease, is frequently an effective parenting strategy. This responsibility may involve remembering to take medication at certain times or reporting back to the parent about any unusual symptoms.

Positive Reinforcement

Positive reinforcement through encouragement and by providing small inexpensive rewards, such as stickers, can be helpful in keeping the child interested and active in disease management. Ultimately, you hope your child takes on these roles without these rewards by realizing that being proactive works well in management of the disease.

Adolescence

The relationship between a parent and a child changes considerably, and may become more challenging in the face of a chronic disorder, as the child enters adolescence. In adolescence, the importance of family relationships may diminish while the importance of friends and peers increases. When adolescents have IBD, the natural tendency of parents to be closely involved in their care may fly in the face of their desire to become more independent. This can be a source of tension between parent and child.

The adolescent may use the management of the disease as a means of asserting independence, sometimes with negative effects when, for example, asserting one's independence means not taking prescribed medications (or not telling parents whether the medication has been taken), not being open about symptoms, and not attending appointments with doctors. There is no easy solution to this problem, but when it occurs,

---

Psychological Growth and Development

IBD should not be allowed to get in the way of your child's normal emotional and psychological growth, including the gradual development of independence from the family and the confidence that goes along with that independence.

Embarrassment

Beyond being painful and uncomfortable, inflammatory bowel disease symptoms may also be embarrassing. To adolescents, for whom image among their peers is often critically important, the embarrassment of the symptoms may be worse than pain or discomfort.

---

these acts of rebellion tend to be part of a larger pattern of independent behavior. Approaching the overall situation rather than specifically focusing on the disease and its management may be an effective way of improving cooperation.

Adolescents may also become angry and frustrated with the disease — the symptoms, the examinations, the medications, and the occasional hospitalizations. Just when they are trying to be like their friends, the disease reminds them that they are, in some ways, different. In addition, the flares of disease and the associated symptoms may get in the way of their ability to attend school regularly and to take part in typical adolescent social and leisure time activities — sports, parties, dating, or just hanging out with friends. Although it may sometimes be difficult to connect with an adolescent, parents, teachers, and friends can all help at these trying times.

Prospects

During the past few decades, inflammatory bowel disease has become more familiar to primary care physicians and pediatricians. As a result, a diagnosis of IBD is usually made early on and is reasonably accurate by using a combination of investigations, such as blood tests, imaging studies, endoscopy, and biopsies.

Although there is no cure for Crohn's disease or ulcerative colitis, once the diagnosis has been made, nutritional counseling, psychological support, drug therapy, and surgery can all help in the right circumstances.

Research continues into the causes of IBD, and breakthroughs, such as the identification of the first Crohn's disease susceptibility gene, provide hope that the causes will be identified and that preventive strategies can be employed in individuals at risk of developing IBD. In addition, the development of new biologic therapies that are founded on advances in research into the altered immune response hold out the hope for newer, more effective therapies over the coming years.

In the meantime, close cooperation between the IBD sufferer and the health-care team provides the best opportunity for effective management of these chronic diseases. This book offers a foundation for that cooperation by providing patients, families, and health-care providers with practical information to assist them in making informed recommendations and decisions.

> **Realistic Expectations**
>
> Be sure to set realistic expectations about the course of the disease, since even with the best management and adherence to medications, disease flares and hospitalizations can occur. This should not be viewed as a failure of either the parents or the child.

Resources and References

Associations and Agencies

Atlas of Inflammatory Bowel Disease

www.endoatlas.com/atlas_ib.html

Features pictures taken during colonoscopy or gastroscopy of areas of the gastrointestinal tract affected by Crohn's disease and ulcerative colitis.

Gastrointestinal Society:
Canadian Society of Intestinal Research

231-3665 Kingsway, Vancouver, BC V5R 5W2
Tel: 1-866-600-4875 (toll-free in Canada)
Email: info@badgut.org
www.badgut.org

A registered charity that works to increase awareness, provides free educational materials to patients and health professionals, and funds medical research in the area of digestive diseases and disorders.

ClinicalTrials.gov

www.clinicaltrials.gov/ct/search?term=inflammatory+bowel+disease

Features the U.S. National Institutes of Health list of all registered clinical trials in inflammatory bowel disease in the United States, Canada, and elsewhere.

Cochrane Collaboration

www.cochrane.org

The Cochrane Collaboration is an organization dedicated to collecting and synthesizing all of the available research data on a wide variety of health-care interventions so that evidence-based recommendations for treatment can be made.

Crohn's and Colitis Foundation

733 Third Avenue, Suite 510, New York, NY 10017
Tel: 1-800-932-2423
Email: info@crohnscolitisfoundation.org
www.crohnscolitisfoundation.org

This foundation supports research in inflammatory bowel disease and also provides educational support for patients and families.

Crohn's and Colitis Canada

600-60 St. Clair Avenue East, Toronto, ON M4T 1N5
Tel: 1-800-387-1479
www.crohnsandcolitis.ca

This patient-founded organization is dedicated to finding the cure for IBD and features an online forum for frequently asked questions and "Ask the Doctor" questions.

U.S. Food and Drug Administration—Center for Food Safety and Applied Nutrition

www.fda.gov/AboutFDA/CentersOffices/OfficeofFoods/CFSAN/default.htm

An excellent American resource on food safety and labeling, as well as links to several useful publications.

Health Canada — Food and Nutrition

www.hc-sc.gc.ca/fn-an/index-eng.php

An excellent Canadian resource on food safety and labeling, as well as links to several useful publications.

Mount Sinai Hospital Inflammatory Bowel Disease Group

600 University Avenue, Toronto, ON M5G 1X5
www.zanecohencentre.com/ibd

The multidisciplinary Mount Sinai Hospital IBD Group in Toronto provides information for patients, health-care providers, and researchers, including two videos — one on life after a stoma and the other on the pelvic pouch procedure.

National Digestive Diseases Information Clearinghouse

2 Information Way, Bethesda, MD 20892–3570
Tel: 1-800-891-5389 Fax: 703-738-4929
Email: nddic@info.niddk.nih.gov
www.digestive.niddk.nih.gov

Information-dissemination service with general information about various digestive diseases, including Crohn's disease and ulcerative colitis.

Ontario Human Rights Commission — Employment

www.ohrc.on.ca/en/issues/employment

This site describes your rights as a prospective employee in the province of Ontario, which may be applicable to other jurisdictions in North America.

United Ostomy Associations of America

P.O. Box 525, Kennebunk, ME 04043-0525
Tel: 1-800-826-0826
Email: info@ostomy.org
www.ostomy.org

This network for bowel diversion support groups in the United States benefits people who have had intestinal diversions and their caregivers. It also includes groups for people who have had urinary diversion procedures.

Ostomy Canada Association

5800 Ambler Drive, Suite 210, Mississauga, ON L4W 4J4
Tel: 1-888-969-9698
www.ostomycanada.ca

This volunteer-based organization provides emotional support, as well as instructional and information services, to individuals who have had intestinal diversion procedures and to their caregivers.

Resource Books for Patients

If This Is a Test, Have I Passed Yet?
Living with Inflammatory Bowel Disease
by Ferne Sherkin-Langer (Fern Publications, 1994)

This is a friendly and useful firsthand account of what it is like to live with IBD and some strategies that proved to be useful.

Learning Sickness: A Year with Crohn's Disease
By James M. Lang (Capital Books, 2005)

This is an account of a year in the life of a man who finally has to come to accept that his Crohn's disease is a part of his life and requires special care.

Sick and Tired of Feeling Sick and Tired:
Living with Invisible Chronic Illness
By Paul J. Donoghue and Mary E. Siegel (W.W. Norton, 2000)

A more thorough overview of the issues of living with an invisible illness by two psychologists.

Codeine Diary: True Confessions of a Reckless Hemophiliac
By Tom Andrews (Harvest Books, 1999)

This is not a book about IBD, but about living with hemophilia. Still, it is a very well-written account of many experiences living with a chronic disease that will be familiar to those with Crohn's disease or ulcerative colitis.

Always Change a Losing Game:
Playing at Life to Be the Best You Can Be
By David Posen (Firefly Books, 1997)
Includes several sensible approaches to stress reduction.

The Feeling Good Handbook
By David D. Burns (Plume, 1999)
This well-written self-help book introduces the techniques of cognitive-behavioral therapy for depression and includes homework exercises.

Full Catastrophe Living: Using the Wisdom of Your
Body and Mind to Face Stress, Pain, and Illness
By Jon Kabat-Zinn (Delta, 1990)
Meditation techniques for stress reduction and health.

Medical Texts
and Journal Articles

American Society for Gastrointestinal Endoscopy Standards of Practice Committee, Shergill AK, Lightdale JR et al. The role of endoscopy in inflammatory bowel disease. Gastrointest Endosc 2015;81(5):1101-21.e1-13.

Bitton A, Buie D, Enns R et al. Treatment of hospitalized adult patients with severe ulcerative colitis: Toronto consensus statements. Am J Gastroenterol 2012;107(2):179-94.

Bressler B, Marshall JK, Bernstein CN et al. Clinical practice guidelines for the medical management of nonhospitalized ulcerative colitis: The Toronto consensus. Gastroenterology 2015;148(5):1035-58.e3.

Candy S, Wright J, Gerber M et al. A controlled double blind study of azathioprine in the management of Crohn's disease. Gut 1995;37(5):674-78.

Casillas S, Delaney CP. Laparoscopic surgery for inflammatory bowel disease. Dig Surg 2005;22(3):135-42.

Colombel JF, Panaccione R, Bossuyt P et al. Effect of tight control management on Crohn's disease (CALM): A multicentre, randomised, controlled phase 3 trial. Lancet. 2018;390(10114):2779-89.

Colombel JF, Sandborn WJ, Reinisch W et al. Infliximab, azathioprine, or combination therapy for Crohn's disease. N Engl J Med 2010;362(15):1383-95.

Colombel JF, Sandborn WJ, Rutgeerts P et al. Adalimumab for maintenance of clinical response and remission in patients with Crohn's disease: The CHARM trial. Gastroenterology 2007;132(1):52-65.

Duchmann R, Kaiser I, Hermann E et al. Tolerance exists towards resident intestinal flora but is broken in active inflammatory bowel disease (IBD). Clin Exp Immunol 1995;102(3):448-55.

Ekbom A, Helmick C, Zack M et al. Ulcerative colitis and colorectal cancer. A population-based study. N Engl J Med 1990;323(18):1228-33.

Elson CO, Cong Y. Understanding immune-microbial homeostasis in intestine. Immunol Res 2002;26(1-3):87-94.

Farmer RG, Whelan G, Fazio VW. Long-term follow-up of patients with Crohn's disease. Relationship between the clinical pattern and prognosis. Gastroenterology 1985;88(6):1818-25.

Feagan BG. Maintenance therapy for inflammatory bowel disease. Am J Gastroenterol 2003;98(Suppl 12):S6-S17.

Feagan BG, Rochon J, Fedorak RN et al. Methotrexate for the treatment of Crohn's disease. The North American Crohn's Study Group Investigators. N Engl J Med 1995;332(5):292-97.

Feagan BG, Rutgeerts P, Sands BE et al. Vedolizumab as induction and maintenance therapy for ulcerative colitis. N Engl J Med 2013;369(8):699-710.

Feagan BG, Sandborn WJ, Gasink C et al. Ustekinumab as induction and maintenance therapy for Crohn's disease. N Engl J Med 2016;375(20):1946-60.

Fefferman DS, Farrell RJ. Endoscopy in inflammatory bowel disease: Indications, surveillance, and use in clinical practice. Clin Gastroenterol Hepatol 2005;3(1):11-24.

Geboes K, De Hertogh G. Indeterminate colitis. Inflamm Bowel Dis 2003;9(5):324-31.

Gillen CD, Walmsley RS, Prior P et al. Ulcerative colitis and Crohn's disease: A comparison of the colorectal cancer risk in extensive colitis. Gut 1994;35(11):1590-92.

Gionchetti P, Rizzello F, Helwig U et al. Prophylaxis of pouchitis onset with probiotic therapy: A double-blind, placebo-controlled trial. Gastroenterology 2003;124(5):1202-09.

Grand DJ, Guglielmo FF, Al-Hawary MM. MR enterography in Crohn's disease: Current consensus on optimal imaging technique and future advances from the SAR Crohn's disease-focused panel. Abdom Imaging 2015;40(5):953-64.

Greenberg GR, Feagan BG, Martin F et al. Oral budesonide for active Crohn's disease. Canadian Inflammatory Bowel Disease Study Group. N Engl J Med 1994;331(13):836-41.

Griffiths AM, Ohlsson A, Sherman PM et al. Meta-analysis of enteral nutrition as a primary treatment of active Crohn's disease. Gastroenterology 1995;108(4):1056-67.

Hanauer SB, Feagan BG, Lichtenstein GR et al. Maintenance infliximab for Crohn's disease: The ACCENT I randomised trial. Lancet 2002;359(9317):1541-49.

Järnerot G, Hertervig E, Friis-Liby I et al. Infliximab as rescue therapy in severe to moderately severe ulcerative colitis: A randomized, placebo-controlled study. Gastroenterology 2005;128(7):1805-11.

Johnson GJ, Cosnes J, Mansfield JC. Review article: Smoking cessation as primary therapy to modify the course of Crohn's disease. Aliment Pharmacol Ther 2005;21(8):921-31.

Khanna R, Bressler B, Levesque BG et al. Early combined immunosuppression for the management of Crohn's disease (REACT): A cluster randomised controlled trial. Lancet 2015;386(10006):1825-34.

Kornbluth A, Legnani P, Lewis BS. Video capsule endoscopy in inflammatory bowel disease: Past, present, and future. Inflamm Bowel Dis 2004;10(3):278-85.

Kruis W. Review article: Antibiotics and probiotics in inflammatory bowel disease. Aliment Pharmacol Ther 2004;20 (Suppl 4):75-78.

Laine L, Kaltenbach T, Barkun A et al. SCENIC international consensus statement on surveillance and management of dysplasia in inflammatory bowel disease. Gastrointest Endosc 2015;81(3):489-501.e26.

Lee J, Allen R, Ashley S et al. British Dietetic Association evidence-based guidelines for the dietary management of Crohn's disease in adults. J Hum Nutr Diet 2014;27(3):207-18.

Löfberg R, Danielsson A, Salde L. Oral budesonide in active Crohn's disease. Aliment Pharmacol Ther 1993;7(6):611-16.

Loftus EVJ, Silverstein MD, Sandborn WJ et al. Crohn's disease in Olmsted County, Minnesota, 1940-1993: Incidence, prevalence, and survival. Gastroenterology 1998;114(6):1161-68.

Markowitz J, Grancher K, Kohn N et al. A multicenter trial of 6-mercaptopurine and prednisone in children with newly diagnosed Crohn's disease. Gastroenterology 2000;119(4):895-902.

Maunder RG. Evidence that stress contributes to inflammatory bowel disease: Evaluation, synthesis, and future directions. Inflamm Bowel Dis 2005;11(6):600-08.

Mawdsley JE, Rampton DS. Psychological stress in IBD: New insights into pathogenic and therapeutic implications. Gut 2005; 54(10):1481-91.

McDonald JWD, Burroughs AK, Feagan BG (eds.). Evidence-Based Gastroenterology and Hepatology, 2nd edition. Oxford, UK: Blackwell Publishing, 2004.

McLeod RS. Surgery for inflammatory bowel diseases. Dig Dis 2003;21(2):168-79.

Munkholm P, Langholz E, Davidsen M et al. Frequency of glucocorticoid resistance and dependency in Crohn's disease. Gut 1994;35(3):360-62.

Narula N, Kassam Z, Yuan Y et al. Systematic review and meta-analysis: Fecal microbiota transplantation for treatment of active ulcerative colitis. Inflamm Bowel Dis 2017;23(10):1702-09.

Peyrin-Biroulet L, Sandborn W, Sands BE et al. Selecting therapeutic targets in inflammatory bowel disease (STRIDE): Determining therapeutic goals for treat-to-target. Am J Gastroenterol 2015;110(9):1324-38.

Ruemmele FM, Veres G, Kolho KL et al. Consensus guidelines of ECCO/ESPGHAN on the medical management of pediatric Crohn's disease. J Crohn's Colitis 2014;8(10):1179-207.

Sandborn WJ, Feagan BG, Rutgeerts P et al. Vedolizumab as induction and maintenance therapy for Crohn's disease. N Engl J Med 2013;369(8):711-21.

Sandborn WJ, Su C, Sands BE et al. Tofacitinib as induction and maintenance therapy for ulcerative colitis. N Engl J Med 2017;376(18):1723-36.

Sands BE, Anderson FH, Bernstein CN et al. Infliximab maintenance therapy for fistulizing Crohn's disease. N Engl J Med 2004;350(9):876-85.

Sartor RB, Sandborn W (eds.). Kirsner's Inflammatory Bowel Diseases, 6th edition. Philadelphia, PA: WB Saunders, 2004.

Satsangi J, Sutherland LR. (eds.). Inflammatory Bowel Diseases. Philadelphia, PA: Elsevier Limited, 2004.

Schwartz DA, Ghazi LJ, Regueiro M et al. Guidelines for the multidisciplinary management of Crohn's perianal fistulas: Summary statement. Inflamm Bowel Dis 2015;21(4):723-30.

Shen B, Fazio VW, Remzi FH et al. Clinical approach to diseases of ileal pouch-anal anastomosis. Am J Gastroenterol 2005;100(12): 2796-807.

Sutherland LR, May GR, Shaffer EA. Sulfasalazine revisited: A meta-analysis of 5-aminosalicylic acid in the treatment of ulcerative colitis. Ann Intern Med 1993;118(7):540-49.

Library and Archives Canada Cataloguing in Publication

Steinhart, Allan Hillary, 1959-, author
    Crohn's & colitis : understanding & managing IBD / Dr. A. Hillary Steinhart, MD, MSc, FRCP(C), Medical Director, Mount Sinai Hospital, Inflammatory Bowel Disease Centre. — Third edition.

Includes bibliographical references and index.
ISBN 978-0-7788-0619-6 (softcover)

    1. Crohn's disease. 2. Ulcerative colitis. I. Title. II. Title: Crohn's and colitis.

RC862.E52S74 2018   616.3'44   C2018-903343-6

Index

A

abscesses, 23, 39, 231
  defined, 12, 42
  detecting, 48, 49, 229
  illustrated, 24, 26, 43, 225
  surgery for, 225, 230, 231, 232
absorption, 12
accelerated step care, 157
acetaminophen (Tylenol), 162
acupuncture, 208
adalimumab (Humira), 191, 197–98
  for Crohn's disease, 193
  and pregnancy, 196
  for skin lesions, 29, 30
adaptable style, 141, 142
adolescents, 244–45. *See also*
    children
  delayed puberty in, 238, 242–43
  education concerns, 62–63
  low bone density in, 31–32
  parenting, 244–45
alcohol (beverage), 123
alendronate, 174–75
anastomosis, 224, 226. *See also*
    pelvic pouch procedure
anemia, 38, 113
ankylosing spondylitis, 28
anorexia, 96, 97. *See also* diet
antibiotics, 81, 89, 163, 179–81. *See*
    also specific drugs
  for Crohn's disease, 160, 179, 235
  for pouchitis, 222
antibodies
  against infliximab, 193–95
  tests for, 45–46
antidepressants, 137, 139
antioxidants, 133
antitumor necrosis factor (anti-TNF),
    29, 30. *See also* adalimumab;
    infliximab
anus, 12, 21, 27, 43. *See also* perianal
    area

arthritis, 28, 162, 175. *See also* joints
5-ASA. *See* mesalamine medications
Asacol (5-ASA), 165
ASCA (anti-Saccharomyces cerevisiae
    antibody), 45
Asians, 15, 105
Aspirin. *See* NSAIDs
avascular necrosis, 175
azathioprine (Imuran), 88,
    132, 181–85, 235. *See also*
    immunosuppressants
  side effects, 158, 243
Azulfidine (sulfasalazine), 164–65

B

bacteria
  Clostridium difficile, 77, 180
  as disease cause, 76–77
  immune response to, 80
  intestinal, 89, 129–30, 202–4
balsalazide (Colazide), 167
behavior, 140–47
  information-gathering styles,
    143–44
  interpersonal styles, 141–43
betamethasone (Betnesol), 177
beverages, 117, 119, 123. *See also* fluids;
    specific beverages
bile, 20
biologic drugs, 163, 190–202. *See also*
    specific drugs
  biosimilars (copies), 200–202
  for children, 241–42
  and pregnancy, 196
  side effects, 193, 195–97
biopsies, 54–55
bisphosphonates, 174–75
bleeding, 36
  medications as cause, 162, 183
blockages. *See* bowel obstruction

medications, 155, 176–77, 179–80, 231, 235
  misdiagnosis of, 227–29
  nutritional therapy, 117
  recurrence, 222–23, 234–35
  in siblings, 74, 84
  smoking and, 14, 66–67, 235
  support resources, 147
  surgical procedures, 222–36
  symptoms, 22–23, 39, 42–43
  treatment goals, 154
cyclosporine, 176, 187–88
cytokines, 38

D

dairy products, 106, 109, 122.
    See also lactose intolerance
dehydration, 125, 217. *See also*
    electrolytes; fluids
Demerol (meperidine), 162
depression, 137–40
diabetes, 174
diarrhea, 38, 43
  dietary management of, 121–23
  medications for, 70, 123–24
  traveler's, 72–73
diclofenac. *See* NSAIDs
diet, 92–133. *See also* nutrition;
    supplements
  advice sources, 93, 98–101, 114, 133
  anti-inflammatory, 132, 133
  elimination/exclusion, 103–4
  fiber in, 118–22
  fluids as, 124–26
  fluids in, 71, 123, 217
  food fears, 127
  high-stool-output management, 121–23
  as IBD cause, 79–80, 92
  individualized, 95
  lactose-restricted, 104–7
  low-fiber, 118–21
  modifying, 102–3, 127
  strictures and, 25
  travel and, 71

dietitians, 93
Dipentum (olsalazine), 168
distension, 12. *See also* gas
doctors. *See* health-care team
double-balloon enteroscopy (DBE), 54
drug therapy. *See also* medications
  approaches to, 156–57
  options for, 160–61
duodenum, 12. *See also* small intestine
dysplasia, 33

E

E. coli Nissle, 203
education, 62–63
electrolytes, 113, 125–26
  ileostomy and, 217
employment, 62, 63–64
endoscopy, 50–54
enemas
  diagnostic, 47
  mesalamine (5-ASA), 168–70
  steroid, 177
energy drinks, 123
enteroscopy, 54
Entocort (budesonide), 152, 176–77
Entyvio (vedolizumab), 198–99, 242
enzymes, 12
  as supplements, 108
  TPMT (thiopurine methyl transferase), 88, 184
episiotomy, 69
erythema nodosum, 29, 237
esophagus, 17
etidronate, 174–75
eye inflammations, 28

F

fat (dietary), 113, 122. *See also* fatty acids
  in immunonutrition, 130–31
fatigue, 38, 43, 66
fatty acids
  essential (omega-3/6), 130–31
  short-chain (SCFAs), 119, 129
fecal microbial transplantation (FMT), 203–4

Imodium, 70, 124

Imuran. *See* azathioprine

incontinence (fecal), 12, 20, 21, 230, 232

    travel and, 70

infections, 26

    biologic drugs and, 195

    as IBD cause, 76–78

    immunosuppressants and, 88, 158, 181, 183–84, 188

    as pelvic pouch complication, 221

infertility, 67

    as medication side effect, 164, 165

inflammation. *See also* immune system

    in gastrointestinal tract, 21–23, 153–54

    of joints, 28

    omega-3 fats and, 130–31

inflammatory bowel disease (IBD), 10–11, 13. *See also* Crohn's disease; ulcerative colitis

    causal factors, 75–89, 92

    complications, 23–33, 48

    coping strategies, 140–48

    diagnosis of, 44–55

    dietary strategies for, 92–133

    as disability, 62, 63–64

    disclosing, 62, 63, 217

    drug therapy for, 87, 152–210

    environmental factors, 78–81, 88–89

    extra-intestinal manifestations, 28–33, 43

    family risk, 74, 82–86

    flares of, 35, 59–60, 69, 153

    gender and, 14

    genetic factors, 81–88

    infection and, 76–78

    information sources, 143, 147–48

    lifestyle factors, 66–67

    onset, 14, 44, 59

    populations affected, 14–15, 105

    prognosis, 57–61

    psychological factors, 80, 134–49, 243–45

    reactions to diagnosis of, 56–57

    remission of, 61, 153

    risk factors, 58–59, 82, 84–85

    support sources, 145–48, 151, 246–49

    surgery for, 65, 67, 211–37

    symptoms, 34–44, 60

    technical terms, 12–13

    treatment goals, 152–54

    treatments for, 61

    of undetermined type (IBDU), 23

Inflectra, 201

infliximab (Remicade), 190, 191–97

    after surgery, 235

    for Crohn's disease, 182, 235

    plus biologic drugs, 182, 186

    and pregnancy, 196

    as rescue therapy, 176

    safety issues, 195–97

    for skin lesions, 29, 30

information

    gathering, 143–44

    sources of, 158–60

interleukin-12/-23 inhibitors, 199–200

Internet, 143, 148, 246–48

interpersonal style, 141–43

intestines. *See* colon; small intestine

inulin, 129

IPAA (ileal pouch-anal anastomosis). *See* pelvic pouch procedure

iron (dietary), 113

irritable bowel syndrome (IBS), 11, 13

J

JAK (Janus kinase) inhibitors, 189–90

Japan, 15, 79

jaundice, 30

jejunum, 13. *See also* small intestine

Jews, 15, 105

jobs, 62, 63–64

Johne's disease, 77

joints, 28, 175

juices, 110, 112, 119, 122. *See also* fluids

MyPlate Food Guidance System
(USDA), 100, 102, 114

N

naproxen. *See* NSAIDs
narcotics, 162
necrosis, avascular, 175
Neoral (oral cyclosporine), 187
nicotine, 14, 67. *See also* smoking
NOD-2 (CARD15) gene, 83
NSAIDs (non-steroidal anti-
inflammatory drugs), 81, 161–62
nurses. *See* health-care team
nutrients, 113, 116. *See also* nutrition;
specific nutrients
absorption of, 12, 17, 18, 20, 108, 112
deficiencies in, 31, 43, 66, 113
as supplements, 108, 109–11, 112–17,
118
nutrition, 31. *See also* diet;
malnutrition; nutrients
for children, 117, 125, 127–28, 238
intravenous, 96, 128, 223
research on, 129–33
support methods, 127–28

O

oat bran, 120–21
olsalazine (Dipentum), 168
omega-3 fatty acids, 130–31
opioids, 162
oral rehydration solutions (ORS), 123,
125
osteoporosis, 31–32
steroids as cause, 31–32, 174–75
ostomy, 71. *See also* colostomy;
ileostomy; stoma
oxycodone, 162

P

pain
abdominal, 37, 38, 42
chronic, 150–51
from fistula, 27
treatment of, 162
pamidronate, 175
pANCA (perinuclear antineutrophil
cytoplasmic antibody), 45–46
pancolitis, 13, 22
pancreas, 20, 183
paramyxoviruses, 78
pelvic pouch procedure, 218–22,
227–29. *See also* pouchitis
complications, 221–22
living with, 220
and pregnancy, 236
Pentasa (5-ASA), 165
perforation, 13
perianal area. *See also* anus
fistulas in, 27
surgery for, 225, 229, 230–33
peristalsis, 13
peritonitis, 26
pharmacogenomics, 87–88
PICC line, 128
PillCam (wireless capsule endoscopy),
53
pneumonia (allergic), 186
pollutants, 80–81
Polycose, 117
population studies, 14–15, 79
potassium, 113, 126
pouchitis, 130, 203, 221–22. *See also*
pelvic pouch procedure
prebiotics, 129
prednisone, 171–75, 211. *See also*
steroids
and supplementation, 112
pregnancy, 67–69
flares during, 69
medications and, 68, 175, 182, 196
steroids and, 68, 175
surgery and, 67, 236
primary sclerosing cholangitis (PSC),
30–31, 32
probiotics, 129–30, 202–3, 222
proctitis, 13, 22, 170, 177. *See also*
ulcerative colitis
proctocolectomy, 227. *See also*
colectomy